DreamBirth

DreamBirth

TRANSFORMING *the* JOURNEY *of* CHILDBIRTH *through* IMAGERY

Catherine Shainberg, PhD

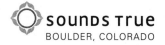

sounds true
BOULDER, COLORADO

Sounds True, Inc.
Boulder, CO 80306

Copyright © 2014 Catherine Shainberg

Sounds True is a trademark of Sounds True, Inc.

DreamBirth® is a registered trademark of Catherine Shainberg.

All names used throughout the book have been changed to protect patients' privacy.

The instruction presented herein is in no way intended to be a substitute for professional assistance such as psychotherapy, counseling, or medical advice.

Published 2014

Cover and book design by Rachael Murray

Cover photo © Nicole Smith, nicolesmithphotography.com

Printed in the United States of America

Library of Congress Cataloging-in-Publication Data

Shainberg, Catherine.

Dreambirth : transforming the journey of childbirth through imagery /
Catherine Shainberg, PhD.

  pages cm

Includes bibliographical references.

ISBN 978-1-62203-090-3

1. Childbirth—Popular works. 2. Pregnancy—Psychological aspects.
3. Dreams—Therapeutic use. 4. Imagery (Psychology)—Therapeutic use.
I. Title. II. Title: Dream birth.

RG661.S47 2013

618.4—dc23

                    2013022062

Ebook ISBN 978-1-62203-164-1

10 9 8 7 6 5 4 3 2 1

For my son, Sam

Imagination is not the talent of some men, but is the health of every man.

RALPH WALDO EMERSON

CONTENTS

Preface . . . ix

INTRODUCTION The Power of Dreaming . . . xvii

PART 1 The Journey of Conception

CHAPTER 1 Pre-conception: Clearing the Way . . . 3

CHAPTER 2 Conception: Calling Forth a Soul . . . 35

PART 2 Milestones of Pregnancy

CHAPTER 3 First Trimester: Exciting News . . . 57

CHAPTER 4 Second Trimester: Basking in the Glow . . . 81

CHAPTER 5 Pregnancy: The Rush to Prepare . . . 115

PART 3 Welcoming Your Baby

CHAPTER 6 Labor: The Flower Opens . . . 153

CHAPTER 7 Postpartum and Bonding: First Smiles . . . 189

PART 4 Embracing the Larger Family

CHAPTER 8 Fathers and Partners . . . 237

EPILOGUE When Your Child Dreams You . . . 271

Excerpts of DreamBirth Stories,
by Claudia Rosenhouse-Raiken . . . 277

Acknowledgments . . . 285

APPENDIX 1 For Surgical Procedures and Medical Tests . . . 287

APPENDIX 2 To Stop Premature Contractions
and Repair Placenta Previa . . . 293

APPENDIX 3 List of Exercises . . . 297

Notes . . . 303

Index . . . 305

About the Author . . . 321

Doulas . . . 323

PREFACE

If I create from the heart, nearly everything
works; if from the head, almost nothing.

MARC CHAGALL

THE NURSE CAME out into the empty waiting room and told me I was pregnant. I had come in for a menopausal test. She showed me the blue dot at the bottom of the cup I had peed in and said this meant a baby was growing in me. I sobbed loudly and for a long time. I couldn't believe it. I was forty-one.

When I finally opened my eyes, the whole room was suffused with soft light. Was it the sun or my emotions? This miracle had happened to me! The shock of amazement stayed with me all through my pregnancy, coloring my every thought and move. Joy grew into a torrent of love and gratitude when I set eyes on my son's face for the first time and held him in my arms, and then later as I watched him grow.

I knew next to nothing about the realities of pregnancy, and my mother and my teacher were far away. So I stocked up on books. I devoured everything I could find, feeding on the clinical facts of a pregnancy and what to expect when labor starts. But there was no book to guide me through the surge of emotions that was shaking me, no dreaming map to this new land I was growing within me, no voice I could hang on to that could lead me down the spiraling path as I searched to connect with my baby using my words and my imagination.

I had so many questions. Could he hear me? Did he feel my love and care for him? Was he developing correctly? Was he protected from the noise and agitation that surrounded me? Was he discovering himself, curled into himself and tucked under my heart? Would he like me, and would I like him? How could I sense, see, and know this stranger growing inside of me?

As my pregnancy progressed, I began to develop my own language of communication. I spoke to my baby endlessly in words, and I sent him images I saw in my mind's eye. I dreamed of him at night and daydreamed about him during the day. I sang him songs; I gurgled and hummed. I stroked my full belly to soothe him when I thought some disruption had upset him. I showed him how he would slide down the birthing canal—which I visualized as the stem of a flower that was opening wide to let him through—and be born into his father's arms in a beautiful garden. My outer and inner worlds grew lush with scents and extravagant blooms. I was immersed in dreaming the magical world of baby and me. I was so much in love that no distraction reached me.

Of course, I had always been a dreamer.

The thought of writing a book about the dreaming power of a pregnant mother never occurred to me. I was in my ivory tower exercising my dreaming with my beautiful growing child; nothing and no one else mattered.

So imagine my surprise when, years later, I was approached to start a training group for birth professionals in prenatal and postnatal imagery. I was not so sure about taking on another responsibility. At that point in my life, I hadn't worked in the birthing field at all. My main clients were people searching for themselves and their spiritual path. But the person who asked me, Claudia Raiken, a craniosacral practitioner and doula who was also my student in imagery, assured me that I would not have to do anything to prepare. "Just let them come and ask their questions," she said.

I had helped many women give birth over the years, using a few simple imagery exercises taught me by Colette Aboulker-Muscat, a revered teacher and lineage holder of the Kabbalah of Light, the Sephardic way of dreaming.[1] I combined her imagery exercises with some I had developed for myself when I was pregnant and about to give birth, and others I had created over the years, specifically for body training and physiological problems.

Still, I wondered what I was going to teach this group. Certainly they could learn the simple relaxation exercises. What else could I do for them? I wasn't a midwife or doula and had no experience in the birthing room except for having given birth to my son in 1986. I was soon to be relieved of that worry.

As I was trying to decide whether to start this training group for birth professionals in prenatal and postnatal imagery, an event occurred that left me thrilled and amazed.

I had gone upstate with a friend to pick up an art piece. An antique dealer had just died and we decided to attend the auctioning off of his collection. Toward the end of the event, I suddenly felt the urge to get up and walk among the objects to be sold. In a corner placed on a table among other forgotten pieces was a large beaded doll. I felt compelled to pick her up. The doll was about twenty-seven inches high, done in African beaded work, and had a pouch made of striped fabric, very worn, over her belly. I signaled the auctioneer that I was willing to bid. No one else was interested, so for the paltry sum of twenty dollars, I bought the doll.

When I got home, I set her up in my entrance hall. The very next day a friend dropped by with a guest who, by chance, was a specialist in African art. His reaction was astonishing: "You've got a spirit doll! Impossible! Nobody gets one unless they're meant to. This is a fertility doll, passed on from mother to daughter. It protects the women of the family and their offspring against dangers in childbirth and labor. See, in the pouch, there's the baby!"

I knew then that my dreaming body had led me to the doll. She was not a particularly attractive specimen, but clearly she had been created with powerful intent. I was struck by the serendipity of a fertility doll landing so conveniently in my lap just as I was asking myself if I should tackle the subject of birthing! I felt certain this was a message from the universe and that I would have guidance in creating the work that would help pregnant women around the world visualize perfect births for their babies. I decided to give the class.

Claudia gathered together seven birth professionals, nurses, psychologists and doulas, all women, to begin training with me. One or two dropped out and a couple more joined us. We met every Wednesday for seven years. The process of creating *DreamBirth*® was collaborative. The birth professionals were my guides to what their clients needed. I created the imagery exercises and walked the birth professionals through the images, and they gave me their feedback. When we were satisfied that the exercises were effectively doing what they were meant to do, the professionals took them to their clients. We got more feedback. Without those seven wonderful women, this work would never have been conceived, gestated, and born.

The DreamBirth imagery exercises are short, precise, and effective. They are designed to consciously move the body and/or the emotions to break up entrenched patterns of fear and old belief systems, restore the natural flow of movement in body and mind, boost the immune system, and facilitate an optimum use of natural capabilities. Today we have more than eight hundred exercises designed for every eventuality dealing with the birth process—and the most prominent and frequently practiced of these exercises are featured in this book. While we have not yet been able to set up clinical trials, the circumstantial evidence for DreamBirth's effectiveness in facilitating a satisfying birth experience is overwhelming.

As I write, we are setting up a research project that we hope to test in hospitals. I have no doubt that our research will prove what we see happening every day to the parents and children we work with: an overall enhanced satisfaction with their birthing experience, healthy and contented mothers and babies, and a quick return to health and well-being for those who have experienced medical intervention.

When I was living in Jerusalem, teaching imagery and movement, many of my young women students were getting married and having children. Jerusalem at the time was still a sleepy hillside town, often troubled by political upheavals, but with streets redolent with bougainvillea and jasmine trees. Our pace was slow, contemplative. We were bathed in history and the mystery inherent in the city's seven hills and olive trees, its three great religions entwined like challah strands. Punctuating our days were the church bells, the muezzin's call to the faithful, the dovening (prayers) wafting out of synagogues and homes.

It is said that in Jerusalem the hills touch the sky. We lived in a magical womb, a sacred place of gestation between heaven and earth.

In Jerusalem babies were born easily to their mothers, or at least to the mothers I taught. Labor was short, easy, and natural. The mothers gave birth without apprehension in their homes, in privacy and surrounded by their womenfolk and the midwife.

How it is to give birth in Jerusalem today, I do not know. Stress, fear, and war were always there, but now that Israel is fast becoming a competitive, materialistic, driven society in the mold of the United States, life's tempo has greatly accelerated. All over the world, both our increasing material desires and the threats to our societies and our planet breed moral and emotional degradation. We are no longer so much interested in the individual as in how to profit from him or her. Rampant greed, dissatisfaction, fear, competition, rage, anxiety, impoverishment of human relations, and loss of spirituality are the modern hydra's many heads. With them also comes a loss of meaning and true connection to our bodies. And while not all pregnant women are directly involved in the rat race of modern living, many cannot escape bathing in its nefarious influence. So do the babies, husbands, doctors, midwives, doulas, relatives, and friends. In today's world, women and their partners cannot help but worry about their birthing experiences and the future of their unborn children.

It is fair to say that in most of the civilized world today, birth comes accompanied by heightened stress levels. Women find it harder or simply impossible to set aside time to concentrate on pregnancy and birth. Most rush around until the very last minute trying to balance increasingly burdensome schedules of work and family, while our societies and governments—with a few exceptions such as Denmark—do very little to preserve that sacred time of gestation during which a pregnant woman should be sitting and brooding over her creation, like a hen over her eggs.

Meanwhile, pregnancy and birth have become big business. Women no longer give birth at home with the help of the local midwife. In the United States, 99 percent of women give birth in hospitals, in antiseptic environments, cheated of the privacy, warmth, and compassion so necessary to a woman in labor. Giving birth is no longer a women's business, conducted among women, in a protective, womblike environment.

Childbirth has been co-opted by the medical experts who look upon its different challenges as symptoms to be treated and, if possible, eradicated through medication and/or surgery. Pregnancy and birth are no longer seen or treated as natural events that need our support and encouragement but as forms of disease. Though the medical model has its place and can be necessary at times, it is important to remember that our bodies are made for childbirth and that it is good to follow nature's lead as much as our bodies will allow us. But as our obstetrician—a very competent, likable woman—told my husband and me on our first prenatal visit: "The only civilized way to give birth is with an epidural!" (An epidural anesthesia is a local nerve block inserted via a catheter into the lower back to numb labor pains.) What the doctor wasn't telling us was that any medication will enter the baby's bloodstream as well as the woman's, slowing down the production of oxytocin, the hormone that facilitates labor and birth. Luckily, my husband, himself an MD, jumped to my defense and reminded the doctor that I was the expert when it came to my body.

Childbirth, the peak experience of a woman's life, has lost both its naturalness and its sacredness. In the medical model of childbirth, laboring mothers are strapped to monitors, as if doctors have forgotten the use of their stethoscopes. They are given epidurals as a matter of course, births are induced, and elective or unnecessary cesareans (40 percent of births in the US) are only growing in number. Wards must be kept clean, quiet, and regulated, and natural birth is not encouraged. "Just think of the noise!" a nurse told me when imagining screaming mothers during natural birth. Hospital costs are fast becoming prohibitive. To give birth is an expensive proposition many couples can't cope with. Yet women continue to flock to hospitals, unaware that there are other choices open to them.

Don't get me wrong. I'm not against doctors. I married one, after all. There is no doubt that allopathic medicine has an important role to play in critical care. So let's not throw the baby out with the bathwater. But have we overdone our need for intervention? We know that in modern societies where the role of the midwife is preferred over that of the physician, women and infants fare better. Midwives have always favored letting nature take its course, as long as labor is progressing normally and safely. Holland, where two-thirds of births are attended by midwives, is rated number one in low infant mortality, whereas today the US is rated twenty-ninth. There is an urgent need to reevaluate our priorities.

After all, who is giving birth, the doctor or you? Will you let the doctor tell you how to manage your body? You and your partner have a say in this process, and so does your baby. I am not suggesting that you do away entirely with the doctor—that would be foolish—but that you shift your perspective and connect more deeply to your own experience and wisdom.

Become active in changing the paradigm. Return the power to nature where it belongs. It has created you with the bone structure, the muscles, the hormones, the cells, the intelligence to give birth. Educated and in tune with your inner self and your baby, you will be able to regain control over your own birthing process, and you will know when to give informed consent if ever an intervention is necessary.

You are the creator, the one holding this new creation in your womb. This book was written for you, to free you to become proactive in your own process. The imaginal exercises herein—short, simple, evocative, and even fun—will be your tools for helping you and your baby toward a safe and satisfying birthing experience.

The Power of Dreaming

Only by way of the Image does a person journey.

PSALM 39:6

THINK OF YOURSELF as an artist faced with a blank canvas. The way you put the first dot on the canvas, the way you develop your drawing, refine it, finish it, frame it, expose it to the world, and give it its freedom, this is how you need to think of husbanding your greatest creation, your child.

You are a life creator, godlike in your ability to bring forth new beings "made in your image." You are mother, *Mère,* and as the homonym reveals, also fundamentally connected to *Mer,* the sea; to *Miriam,* prophetess; to *Maria,* mother of god. The relationship among these same-root words suggests that water elicits images and visions, that water is the mother out of which creation emerges, and that creation is an act of love. You too, like a god, can dream the world into being, learn to look into the waters of your body and dream the arc of your movement from conception to motherhood. Dreaming, as I hope to prove to you, is the language of your body.

How do you return to the deep dreaming knowledge and intelligence that are inherent in you? Oral and written testimonies in many traditions point the way. While I will be choosing examples from the

Western spiritual tradition familiar to Christians, Muslims, and Jews alike because that is my tradition, feel free to replace those stories with some from your own tradition. Feel free to substitute the word God with Goddess or Allah or the Divine or simply the Mystery, if that feels more appropriate. I honor, recognize, and welcome the dream stories in all traditions and believe that all the great traditions point to the same truths. Perhaps you don't feel connected to any spiritual tradition. If that is the case, you can connect to nature, to whose laws we are all subject.

In my tradition the most ancient source is the Bible, which has much to teach us about dreaming and childbearing. "Go to your-self!"[2] says God to his prophet on the first leg of Abraham and his wife Sarah's journey from barrenness to triumphant conception and birth. Itzhak—*laughter,* they aptly name their son. We are all spiritual creatures, and for all of us our spiritual roots, I am sure, state it as clearly: you must return to yourself, learn to know yourself and your body, the sacred vessel within which the seed of creativity grows.

As you read these pages you may be thinking that you have already tried everything humanly possible to make your dream come true, but it hasn't. You are still waiting to conceive or to hold on to your babies. You are sad, angry, envious, and discouraged, just like Sarah probably was. To you I say, right from the start, do not lose hope! I have seen miracles. Imagination is a magical tool that has the power to transform your body and your future. You have not yet learned how to work with your images to talk directly to your body. Images are the experiencing language your body understands. Much of your body responds to subconscious programs. The subconscious is like a computer. If infected by a virus—serving up negative belief systems, negative emotional programs, damaged organs, and the like—your subconscious cannot discard it. It will perpetuate the version of your-self containing the virus until you do something to clear out the virus, thus allowing your body to return to a full and healthy functioning version of itself. In the pages that follow, you will learn how to iden-tify those viruses and how to give the subconscious commands that will clear them. After all, Sarah was close to a hundred years old when she conceived. In my practice I have witnessed again and again the power of the imagination to make the impossible come true. Please continue reading. This book is for you too!

WATERS OF THE CREATIVE IMAGINATION

What are these waters of the imagination? We know that without water our planet would be uninhabitable; that we ourselves develop in the slightly saline waters of the amniotic sac; that our bodies are 85 percent water. Looking into clear waters, we see our own image reflected back to us. Water, mirrorlike, supports us in emptying our minds and allows us to see the true images and patterns that float in the deeper recesses of our minds. For this reason, it is the medium most commonly used in divination, the art of seeing the potential future, of looking into the vast emptiness and conceiving newness.

So it is in the waters of your body that you first dream of conceiving and bringing forth. Often called the waters of the unconscious, they are only unconscious because you are not focusing your attention on them. Focusing is all it takes to consciously begin the process of dreaming forth a new life.

All around the *Mare* Mediterranean, from Egypt to Palestine to Greece, to Italy, France, Spain, and North Africa, women used dreaming as their language of choice. Dreaming was an integral process in rituals, mysteries, healings, and procreation. In Egypt the residence of the female goddess of creation, Isis, who protects fertility and motherhood, is surrounded by water. To reach her temple, Philae, women traveled by boat across deep waters. Through water they were induced into the dream state that is at the source of fertility.

Creation or transformative stories generally begin with a vision or a dream. Your imagination, birthed in the waters of the body, is the secret to preparing both your body and your psyche for becoming a happy and successful parent.

We are reminded of the connection between fertility and dreaming through the many ancient records of women's dreams that deal with conception and childbirth. Women's healing dreams are inscribed on the great steles of Delphi in Greece. Women went to Delphi to be healed of barrenness or other womanly disorders by entering into womblike sleep in the Asclepion, the temple room for dream incubation. In their dreams a god appeared to them and showed them the way to fertility.

In spiritual traditions around the world the Divine partners with us in our ability to conceive and bring forth. By contemplating a god's image through the many images that arise within them, women learn to create.

This book is not a how-to about becoming a parent. Rather, it is about imagination and accessing our dreaming power in the creation of new life. It is about restoring the creative act to women and their partners who have lost it to the Western medical model and the belief that we reproduce through genetic accidents.

Where do babies come from? Are we just flesh, and is creating new life, on any level, purely mechanistic? How do cells differentiate to become lungs, heart, kidneys? Does something animate us that we are not taking into account? Is our godlike ability to "make images" involved? And if so, can we harness our imagination?

Can we plunge again into our sea of dreaming and create our babies perfectly, birthing them in exhilaration and with ease?

IMAGINATION

Who are we if not our dreams?

The belief that our bodies have nothing to do with our hopes, aspirations, fears, or guilt has led us to ignore the power of our psyche on the physical. Our psyche—our thoughts, feelings, memories, behaviors, and especially images—filters the way we view reality. I remember a young woman who had been raped subconsciously stopping the birth. Although the doctor said she was ready to push, she couldn't. It was "dirty down there," was her comment. The baby was delivered by Caesarean.

We each live in a personal reality filled with the images of our experiences—past, present, and projected future—whose visions, sounds, scents, taste, and kinesthetic feelings are at the source of our beingness. When I use the word "image" I am referring to the 3-D inner world that we each inhabit, activated by all five of our senses, and that contains our memories, perceptions, responses to outer or inner stimuli, dreams, and creative insights. The word "image" is a convention, used because the visual sense is the most prominent sense for most people and because seeing encompasses the other four senses. Imaging is an embodied experience in which all the senses are in synergy: you can see, smell, hear, taste, and touch in your inner world as vividly as you can in the outer reality.

Our identity—past, present, and future—arises from this field of images, involving bodily movements, sensations, and emotions of which we are hardly aware but which define our lives. Each of us lives in multiple strata, or what I call *dreamfields*™: individual, familial-ancestral, social, national, and global. Unless we explore those dreamfields, discovering in the process what makes us act as we do, we will forever be held back in our ability to expand beyond our current limited span of behaviors.

The dreamfield offers us answers to many questions, and can lead us to what we yearn for. Why, with no medical impediment, are some women fertile and others not? What makes some babies develop perfectly while others struggle? If dreaming is an inherent tool for creativity, if properly channeled can it help us manifest a more wholesome future and happier babies?

Think back: as a small child, did you wonder whether you, like your parents, would have children? As a little girl rocking your doll, speaking softly to her, were you not teaching yourself the gestures, sensations, and feelings of being just like Mom? And your brothers, watching their father being tender or firm with them, were they not bursting with pride at the thought of one day being just like Dad? Or, through disappointment and loneliness, were they settling on the idea that they would become "a dry fruit"—infertile—as one little boy said to his hostile father? Did you conceive the idea that you would not have children because Mom was always so sick, and you promised never again to be a burden? Are you locked into an ancestral belief system—for example, that all the women in your mother's family as far back as memory goes had difficult births—that will dictate your reproductive future?

The point is that for many of us, the idea of having a child is already in gestation years before its manifestation. We will have one boy and two girls, or a third child later on in life, or only girls! On the other hand, we may *know* that we will never have children or that one day we will adopt a little Chinese girl. We long for the accomplishment of some destiny we intuit, or fear the void of some terrible impossibility we divine. Do we know our destiny because it is written in the stars, or do we create it through our dreaming? Are these two, destiny and dreaming, interconnected? If so, can we change our destiny by responding to and engaging with the rich terrain of our dreaming?

DREAMING AS A VERB

Dreaming is a verb that indicates an ongoing flow of action, a progression, and a journey. It is not static. It is important to recognize this quality of dreams because it is this process of dreaming that we are engaging in this book. We usually do not speak of dreaming but of "having dreams." Dreams are what we have at night: "a series of images, ideas and emotions occurring in certain stages of sleep"; or "a daydream, reverie"; or an "aspiration, ambition."[3] What these definitions suggest but neglect to spell out is that we are dreaming all the time. We do not dream just at night. We are accumulating experiences all the time and that is what I call "dreaming." You are dreaming as you read this book. Because the flow of your dreaming is subconscious, part of the right-brain activity that never ceases, you are not generally aware of it. You will become more aware during pregnancy because you are tuned in to yourself and your baby. You will also remember your night dreams more easily. Night dreams are just windows, cutouts, in the flow of your dreaming. You recall them because of their intensity of sensations or emotions, or because they are weird enough to surprise you.

The flow of dreaming, on the other hand, is what the right hemisphere of your brain is engaged in at all times, through neuronal pathways connecting with the older mammalian brain and the much older reptilian brain. At every moment, operating like a giant radar, your brain is assessing where you are spatially and what surrounds you. It is also assessing what is happening inside your body.

Dreaming is instantaneous. It is the way your right brain reads spatial and sensory cues and movements. Your right brain is the screen that picks up signals near and far, transmitted through the receptors of your senses (eyes, ears, nose, tongue, skin), reshaping them into readable images. It is your visual reader. While the spoken or written words that are the language of the left brain take time to digest and comprehend, an image speaks volumes in an instant and effortlessly communicates a multilayered reality.

Dreaming is also interactive, responding or reacting to what it senses and sees. Dreaming is the way your body, having received new information, reorganizes itself in view of this information. Take a look at what this word contains: in *form*. This is the secret of how your right brain works: it recognizes form. It fits one form into another, like the many pieces of a puzzle or like an Escher painting, creating a detailed, precise, and constantly updated mapping of your life. But while the pieces may fit together, sometimes the overall picture doesn't, revealing some fixed pattern in one of your dreamfields. The dreaming will sense that something is blocking the flow and will send up signals: nightmares, repetitive dreams, emotional disturbances, physical pains. What do these signals call for? What do they need you to hear?

Far from being "garbage" that is being purged from your brain at night, as some modern scientists have suggested,[4] your dreams are asking you to deal with the difficulties in their mapping. If you take your dreaming seriously, you will soon see that dreaming is both the diagnosis *and* the cure. The dreaming may show you a dark spot in your stomach. The image works like everyday reality; it has a need. It calls for you to clean the spot. You will be amazed, when you do the exercises, at how effective this simple response to your image is. The language of the body is image-experience. An image pops up on the screen of your right brain, showing you the actual state of your stomach. When you respond to the image by forming an image in your mind's eye of cleaning up the spot, just as you would respond to a stain on your floor by wiping it up, you are actually communicating with your body and it will send the necessary energy flow to help you with your digestion. By responding to your dream images, you are given the opportunity to play with corrective images and actively participate in your own cure. But for most people, everything still happens subconsciously.

What if you were to become aware? Could your dreaming become an instrument in your ambition—a way of channeling your energy, of focusing your intention toward an aspiration? A way, if you harnessed it, of manifesting?

HOMEOSTASIS

The body is an amazing organism. It talks to itself and to the world at large in myriad ways. We are only cognizant of the more gross manners of our interaction: our movements, expressions, exclamations, or words. What happens below the surface or at the deeper strata of our nervous and cellular systems is unknown to us except through our dreams. Generally, the body finds its own balance; it is amazingly wired to maintain a stable, constant condition called homeostasis. In fact, the body's condition is neither stable nor constant but striving at all times to maintain a state of physiological equilibrium, like a nautical compass on rough seas.

States of mind such as worry, frustration, or any other form of unease are signs that the flow of dreaming is somehow impeded. The body is having a hard time finding its equilibrium; homeostasis is compromised. The system is showing signs of strain or of breaking down. Before malaise even appears in your consciousness as unease or disease, your dreaming is registering the strain. Like a subterranean tidal wave, unease moves below the surface of a seemingly calm ocean, taking its time to surface. If you are lucky, some sudden eruption—a night dream or daytime vision—will burst forth like a fish from the deep to alert you. If you pay attention, if you give your dreaming its due and take seriously what it is showing you, you can do something about changing course. Forewarned, you can actively respond to the needs of the images you have had.

Within homeostasis is a natural intent toward which it strives. The intent of the body is like that of a seed that knows itself, knows that it must and will grow roots, trunk, branches, leaves, flowers—always moving toward fulfilling its ultimate purpose to produce fruit. We see the process of homeostasis occurring within the womb as the fetus grows to maturation, at which stage homeostasis dictates the release of the labor phase. Your dreaming shows you all this long before you are aware of outward physical signs. Wouldn't it be advantageous to be forewarned?

The trick, of course, is to become aware of your dreaming—which you have the ability to do.

CONSCIOUS DREAMING

As a child, you were aware of your dreaming. In fact, being less verbal then and therefore less self-reflective, you lived in your dreaming. Your anger was a spitting dragon; your wonder, an angel with gossamer wings. You were the bad guy and, in the next instant, a policeman.

Your play showed you what you felt in the moment as well as how to transform the situation if you needed to.

But this facility was likely bred out of you, and if it was, it is necessary to reacquaint yourself with this childhood language of dreams.

There are two ways to do this: 1) remembering your night dreams and 2) turning your eyes inward to gaze at the *imaginal* field. You may think this is impossible, but if you read on, you'll see it's quite easy. Soon you'll be able to do both quite comfortably.

Once you are aware of your dreaming, you're ready to become an active participant in your own bodily process. *Dreaming is the language your body understands.* Your body shows you in images what it is experiencing, and you can access your body by responding in images. With the subconscious, your language of choice is always images. Using this language, you can participate consciously in what was for you, until now, only a subconscious bodily process. By dialoguing with your body, responding with appropriate images to the images your body shows you, you become a partner in helping it meet its challenges and maximize its performance.

It will no longer be your body doing to you, but you and your body doing together. Think of yourself as the rider, your body as the horse. If you do not learn to engage your horse, you will always remain an unskilled rider, flung about and maybe thrown by a horse you cannot control. Wouldn't you rather be one with your horse?

Conception, pregnancy, and birth can be a smooth or a rocky ride. This book will give you tools to make it a smooth one. Like Olympic athletes who train their bodies by visually rehearsing their moves, you will learn the imagery that will help prepare your body for conception, sustain it through the transformations of pregnancy, and train it for the effort of pushing your baby out. Athletes train to compete. As a future mother, you are preparing to "labor." This word suggests that strong body activity is involved. You can use imagery to become, like an Olympic medalist, champion of your labor.

If you learn to quiet your left brain (the doubting Thomas of your conscious mind) and be wholly involved in your dreaming, you will give birth in a state of peak experience or heightened awareness in which body and mind are experienced as one. This is what athletes call "the zone." If you are completely in your dreaming, what seemed like hard labor can become effortless, ecstatic, and orgasmic.

IMAGES MOVE THE BODY

Every time you create images, you speak to your body. You create images in your night dreams and day dreams, when you paint or sculpt, when you are envisioning a goal, or planning a new venture. You also create images whenever you want to move your body, although you are not generally aware of those. Countless research projects have shown that images affect the body in ways that can be quantified: for example, precise imaging of a physical movement activates the appropriate motor neurons. By visualizing yourself running, you are actually initiating micromovements in your leg muscles. To check this for yourself, imagine tasting a lemon. Does this activate your salivary glands?[5] From mental rehearsal utilized in sports therapy[6] to its applications in weight loss,[7] pain management,[8] healing, psychotherapy,[9] or spiritual development,[10] "images hold enormous potential for healing . . . A large body of recent scientific research on imagery indicates that these claims [for the effectiveness of imagery] are justified."[11] Imagery allows you to speak to even the most subterranean parts of your body.

For the last forty years I have consistently seen beneficial results when using imagery exercises with my clients and students. Facilitating all manner of positive outcomes—relaxation, pain management, physiological changes, reversals of medical complications, and the healing of emotional wounds and trauma—the exercises act like a rehearsal practice for life. They will provide you with the inner strength and stamina you need to face the challenges of becoming a parent.

HOW TO USE THIS BOOK

There are many different approaches to imagery. My own tradition is unique in that it is very quick. The quicker you work, the more instantaneous and true your body response will be. These are not long relaxations or contemplations but a quickening of your body's healthy response. While you will not be lingering over your images—an exercise may take from one to three minutes, maximum—the effect will be deeply powerful, and you will feel as if you had actually been in profound meditation for a long time.

These short inductions allow you to instantly engage your dreaming self and dialogue with it. I use the word "dialogue" with purpose, as the work is not to force the body but to elicit its complicity. The body never lies. You may fantasize but, like the horse, your body will balk. You can only go with the true homeostatic intent of your body. Again, when I speak of body, I am not speaking only of the flesh but of deep embodiment: the five levels of body, spirit, mind, soul, and oneness are all engaged.

While this book contains exercises for every eventuality in the conception, pregnancy, birthing, and postpartum experience, what you will find here are the basic visualizations you and your partner will need to enable your experience to be health enhancing and meaningful. Each exercise is explained, then given. The exercises appear throughout the chapters, highlighted so you can access them easily. It is best to read them and then practice them immediately; you don't want to lose the surprise effect. Imagery exercises should sound like poetry and transport you through your surprise to a heightened state of well-being.

The book is fairly chronological, and instead of beginning with pregnancy, we start in the pre-creation time, which is "pregnant" with possibilities. This is the time when intent and imaging are critical.

The first part of the book, The Journey of Conception, has two chapters, Pre-conception: Clearing the Way and Conception: Calling Forth a Soul. The first deals with the preparation of body, mind, and emotions for conception. Like a good farmer, you will want to clear the land, removing stones and fertilizing your field, before you start planting your seeds. Recognizing the reality of your terrain—engaging your dreaming, creative self toward optimizing your options—is your first step.

The second step is about focusing your body, mind, and heart to call forth a soul: to invite your child into your life. Conscious conception is a labor of love requiring your full attention. Right timing, purity of intent, attention to the enhancement of every sensation, joyous expectation, and bliss: these are the auspicious conditions for attracting into your home a healthy, alert, and peaceful baby.

The second part, Milestones of Pregnancy, is about pregnancy itself—the attitudes, continuing intents, and visualizations needed to bring your child to fruition. You are the farmer watching your plants grow. You have a lot of maintenance, watering, weeding, and troubleshooting to address.

The third part, Welcoming Your Baby, is about giving birth; it prepares you through dream work for labor and prepares those around you to be fully conscious, engaged, and focused on the process of letting nature take her course. All the possible scenarios are addressed in a positive light to enable the experience to be a happy and successful one. This part is also about bonding, lactating, postpartum blues, growing into a parent, and recovering your nonpregnant self.

The fourth part, Embracing the Larger Family, addresses the partners and helpers who want to participate in their own way and within their own levels of comfort. It is also about the new configuration to which partners and family must adjust, and about the possibility of becoming active participants in creating this new configuration.

Each section contains visualizations specifically designed to enhance and facilitate your journey and that of your partner, family, and helpers. The book is presented linearly because you are living through an unfolding process. But remember that your subconscious is not linear.

This means that if you pick up this book when you are already far advanced in your pregnancy, you need not be upset that you didn't get to do the exercises on time. The subconscious—the larger part of you—exists beyond time and space. You can still do the exercises you missed doing before conception or early in your pregnancy. You can even do them after your child is born. You can repair the past by simply doing the appropriate exercises *now*.

The creation process is never ending. We must be aware of both its present and its unfolding, trying not to suppress its different manifestations but graciously and creatively engaging every phase of the journey. How to do this, with ease and happiness, is the subject of the concluding chapter.

Parenting in exuberance requires your full participation and responsiveness. But remember: dreaming is not a chore nor is it work. In fact, to access your dreaming you must relax, empty your mind, and enjoy the show. You will find that practicing your imagery is fun, creative, surprising, and deeply moving. Why not access this amazing tool you have been given?

Please note: I will be using the word "partner" throughout this book, as I welcome all family configurations that wish to enhance their experience of birthing through DreamBirth. To make this an easier read, I have chosen to address the partner as male.

When addressing the child, I have chosen not to alternate the use of gender at each paragraph, as is commonly done in pregnancy books. Instead, I have alternated the gender from chapter to chapter.

While this book seems to address the first-time mother, it is equally beneficial for a second- or third- or fourth-time mom.

Finally, mothers expecting twins can use the exercises the same way any other mother would. Simply visualize both children when doing the exercises.

PART ONE

✥

The Journey
of Conception

I

Clearing the Way

Nothing happens unless first a dream.
CARL SANDBURG

HAVE YOU EVER heard your unborn children calling?

Long before my son was born, I could hear him! You may think me crazy, but there he was, a sweet cherub standing on a fluffy pink cloud in the sky, waving his chubby hand and smiling. "Mom, Mom, are you ready?"

But I wasn't ready. I hadn't yet met my soul mate. And to be honest, I wasn't prepared to give up my all-consuming and precious time with my teacher, Colette. Leaving my spiritual mother to start a family was not on my immediate agenda. Still, my biological clock kept ticking.

Colette had also heard her children calling, as had her mother and grandmother. I was well aware that we may have a destined soul mate or a destined child, but that the choices we make along the way can change our destiny. I accepted that my priorities had changed and that, given the time constraint of my biological clock, I might never become a wife or a mother.

THE WOMAN WHO MAKES BABIES

It is said that in Jerusalem, where I lived at the time, sky and earth meet like a saucepan and its lid. The earthly city is a microcosm of the heavenly one, a mirror image, a map of the celestial qualities it strives to embody. In this cauldron of spirituality, where the three great Western religions vie for room, I had found my own private womb within a womb. To get there, I walked down a long, winding street bordered by a variety of magnificent trees. Hidden among bushes and lilac trees halfway down the street was a little blue gate. Beyond the gate were seven stone steps leading into a garden with a small terrace shaded by a large jasmine tree. Entering my teacher's space felt like returning to the lost garden of Eden. There, I was safe again in metaphorical amniotic waters, cradled by love, listening to words and heartbeats that structured the world for me. My teacher never left her house so I was sure to find her there.

Colette was the last lineage holder of an ancient Sephardic family of Kabbalists. Her work restored receptive, surrendering qualities to women—qualities that are embodied in the word *kabbalah*, which means receiving. She was famous for curing barrenness, whether of mind, heart, or body, and for igniting the creative flow. She was known as "the woman who makes babies."

Closing my eyes at her request, I entered into the womb of my body and, in the dark, discovered the spark of light that begins all creation. From that light unfolded many offshoots of my imagination: wonderful, terrifying, awe-inspiring waking dreams that echoed the dreams I had at night. Was I indulging in fantasies? My family, far away in France, thought so and warned me against dreaming my life away.

But I was mesmerized. I found in those inner images an ever-flowing source of inspiration and joy. When I had first met Colette, my life was in shambles. I had lost all purpose and direction in life. I was closer to despair than I had ever been before. I was sick in body and soul. In one of the first exercises she had me do, she asked me to close my eyes and image catching a ray of light. "Draw a circle in the upper right-hand side of the blue sky. What appears out of the circle?"

I saw coming out of the circle a huge being of light accompanied by thousands of white doves, all flying toward me. The being gave me his name and assured me that I had nothing to fear, that my life's work

4

was beginning. I felt immeasurably comforted and reassured. Meaning and purpose returned to my life. The images sustained and guided me. The more I practiced dreaming, the more grounded I felt, as if my images directly affected my body as well as my soul. For the first time, I had glimpses of feeling united within myself, of becoming a healed and whole being. I began to manifest my creativity. Under Colette's guidance, I gave birth to myself.

CHILDREN OF OUR IMAGINATION

How powerful are these children of our imagination? Are they pure fantasy and, if so, a self-indulgence? How do we know the images from our dreams are actually relevant to our lives and not some random firing of our brains? And is there more to making images than meets the eye?

Today many self-help books incorporate visualizations with other forms of self-care. For the most part, these visualizations are suggested to facilitate relaxation and well-being.

But I was beginning to realize that the images in my mind that Colette's exercises generated were much more than simply agents of relaxation and well-being. Short and jolting to the imagination, they provoked revelations and brought up information I never knew was in me. They showed me talents and abilities I didn't know I had. Where I thought I would never have the courage to go out into the world, to have my own business, to support myself through teaching, to write, my images showed me doing just that. Because I had seen that I could and had experienced what these pursuits meant (albeit only in my imagination), I went out and did it. My images were the messengers and engine of my development. Where there had been darkness, now I was being in-formed and re-formed! I saw transformation in all my bodies— mental, emotional, physical—elevating my spirit to heights I had never envisioned before. Like a seed packed with the potential of its own growth, I felt the darkness in me holding the secret to my embodiment, past and future. I was becoming more vibrant, more alive, more present.

But what exactly had happened? What comes first? Out of the darkness comes the light, and in the light is programmed creation? Or is it that in the triggering of light comes knowledge of selfhood from which our brain, spine, organs, limbs, and every part of ourselves—body, mind, and soul—emerge? I noticed that if I looked back even further, to before I'd met Colette, there were dreams that revealed much of my life's journey. My imagination had always guided me.

SEMINAL DREAM

The long journey toward my child was ignited in my work with Colette but started much earlier when, as a little girl, I imagined my belly swelling my dress. Holding my doll, smiling at her full face, imagining that she was smiling back, I knew I was born to be a mother. I was rehearsing my seminal dream of motherhood as far back as I can remember. Seminal dreams are what propel us forward. We can reject them, think we kill and bury them, but they will come out, showing themselves in clear or twisted ways depending on whether we have chosen to honor or ignore them. So many women are impregnated with this dream of motherhood that we can safely say it is imprinted in our genes. As far back as we can remember, society, our cultural expectations, and our spiritual texts have urged us to "be fruitful and multiply." It is both our nature and our task. Each feeds upon the other to manifest women's inescapable fate: that of furthering our species.

But today that seminal dream has been called into question by a changed sexual context. Scientific breakthroughs in obstetrics and reproductive endocrinology have given us control over our reproductive cycle. Women educated in modern fertility methods need no longer be enslaved to their natural condition as reproductive wombs. We are free to decide when and whether to become pregnant. While this newfound freedom is gratifying, it does put the onus on us to decide whether or not to have children.

Have our priorities shifted? Do we want to have children? It is a question we need to address sooner rather than later. As more and more of us go to college and enter the workforce, our priorities shift and we tend to postpone having children until later in our fertile cycle—with the result that in the US, 20 percent of women ages forty to forty-four have no children, double the rate of thirty years ago, according to the latest Census Bureau report; 27 percent of these women have graduate or professional degrees. We find this trend toward lower birth rates in all the developed countries. While world overpopulation—by the year 2050 we will have grown from an estimated 6.6 billion people to an unbelievable 9.3 billion—is taxing our natural resources to the straining point, first-world countries are battling with decreasing birth rates. Already today in Britain and soon in the US, our birth rate will not be high enough to replenish our dying populations.

The contradictions we endure are further fueled by knowledge of environmental threats, global warming, world hunger, collapsing financial markets, wars, and weapons of mass destruction. Other serious factors are adding to our general malaise about procreation: sperm counts have been falling over the last century (an estimated one in ten men is affected for reasons unknown, although environmental and food pollution is suspected); marriage percentages are in decline; homosexuality is on the rise. We are left to wonder whether we are witnessing an unprecedented evolutionary trend away from the traditional need to "fructify and multiply" toward a need to limit procreation. Is it surprising that, in this atmosphere, the thought of conceiving is fraught with anxiety?

It therefore becomes imperative for us to have a way to silence work and financial pressures long enough to access our inner truth. To become conscious of our true desires and personal seminal dream is not a luxury. Will we allow ourselves to become the victims of fate, manipulated by the pressures and accidents of life, or will we choose our own destiny?

CONSCIOUS CONCEPTION

For some of us, conception just happens. It is an unwanted accident. We accept the irrefutable, or we decide to get rid of the unplanned pregnancy. In either case, we are put on notice that ignorance and lack of awareness are no excuse.

We don't have to be the puppets of fate: we have advantages over previous generations, foolproof tools to prevent or interrupt gestation. Our particular challenge is the freedom to choose conception or avoid it. Should we follow the trend and decide not to have children? Should we risk bringing children into this dangerous new world? Do we have the resources? Will having a child disrupt the lifestyle we are accustomed to? Should we simply put off the decision, with the risk that we will regret our decision if it turns out to be too late? Our freedom to choose does not, of course, guarantee that we will get pregnant. But at least we have the power to become proactive.

Freedom requires much more of us. It is easier to resign ourselves to the vagaries of fate than it is to become our own self-creators. Easier to be told what to do than to take a leading role in the drama of our own lives. The openness of freedom begs the question *What do I really want?* Becoming proactive means becoming conscious of our own inner needs. Is choosing to have a child the right and good thing for me to do now? Is it right for my partner? My family? The need to look within, to wake up to our own personal dream—whether that dream says to conceive, to adopt, or simply to abstain—is paramount. We must open our eyes to our truth and make our decision not based on circumstances or the needs of others but on informed choices. By "in-formed," I mean formed from within! For it is ultimately our dreaming body that tells us what is right for us.

THE STILL SMALL VOICE

The voice of the dreaming body is simple and quiet. In the Bible it is called "the still small voice." It has no drama, no anger. You know it because it doesn't come with a tidal wave of emotion.

"The voice" is not always just a sound. It is often an image. It can also be a smell, taste, touch, or kinesthetic movement. For some, the voice ignites instantaneous change or manifestation. For others, the voice is heard but manifestation lags. Without the perfect vibrational alignment of your whole being with what you are asking for and hearing from the voice, the dream cannot come into reality. More is required.

We need to identify the "voice" among all the other voices competing in our heads. Visually this is akin to when ripples agitate a pond. It can be quite difficult, if not impossible, to see the fish below the surface. To hear or see, we must stop all agitation. When the pond is still, we can see the fish moving, hear the flapping of their tails in the water. When the mind is still, free of clutter, we can begin to hear that one guiding voice.

Like fish, the voice/image must be lured to the surface. The bait here is your question. Without a question, the answer cannot come. For some, the question remains subterranean, never formulated but floating just below the surface. For others, the act of "hovering over the waters" of our chaos and confusion—as God does to bring forth creation—has not even occurred. Learning to become conscious starts here. By asking the question or, if that is too confusing, by asking, "What *is* the question?" you inevitably call for an answer. This is where creativity begins.

REMEMBERING OUR DREAMS

You can take advantage of your dreams starting now. But first there are things you can do to help yourself remember your dreams. Tell yourself that you want to remember your dreams. Share your dreams with your partner upon waking up. When someone else expects you to remember your dream, you will. Immediately upon waking, write down your dream. It is good to have a notebook next to your bed.

REMEMBERING YOUR NIGHT DREAM
exercise I

Go out and buy yourself a blank notebook. Pick a notebook that you love; this is going to be your book to record your dreams. The nicer it is, the more convinced your dreaming will be that you are interested in hearing from it. Bring your notebook home and open it to the first page. Write on it, *Dream Book*. Put it on your nightstand next to your bed. Just before you go to bed, open it to the next page, write at the top of the page that night's date, and then leave the book open and place your pen inside. You have established your intention to remember your dream. As you go to sleep, remind yourself that you want to remember your dream. It is useful at first to remind yourself to wake up at the time you have the dream so you can catch it and write it down when it is fresh in your memory. If this doesn't work for you, write down your dream in the morning. Record everything you remember, even if you think it is not important. Later you will see that your dreams know best what is important. Do the particular task of asking the question—your "bait"—for a week. (Of course, it is good to continue recording your dreams beyond the first week. You will learn so much about yourself if you do.)

The moment you get wrapped up in your day, you become more likely to forget pieces of your dream. So when you wake up in the morning, give yourself a little time before jumping out of bed. Relax in the same posture you were in when you were dreaming. This helps stimulate recall. Write down exactly what you saw, heard, and felt in your dream. If the answer you receive from the dream seems unclear to you, let it resonate in your mind for a few days. Do not try to analyze it. Dreams should not be interpreted but simply felt. Just sit with it like you would a mysterious painting. Soon its meaning will open up to you.

After the week is over and you have managed to write down the dreams you remember, you are ready to ask a question of your dream. Here you are using your conscious mind to focus your dreaming mind. In focusing, you narrow the field of stimuli. You create the window, circumscribe your field of interest. Your dreaming, true to form, will respond to the stimulus.

ASKING A QUESTION OF YOUR NIGHT DREAMS
exercise 2

As you are lying in bed just before going to sleep, limbs uncrossed, eyes closed, breathe out slowly three times, with your mouth slightly open. (Don't worry about breathing in. If you are empty, the breath will fill you.) Count from 3 down to 1, seeing the numbers clearly in your mind as you exhale. Now imagine that as you breathe out once again to zero, the zero appears as a circle of light in front of your eyes. Imagine writing your question within the circumference of the circle. Make the question simple, direct, and short.

Your attitude behind your question is important. If you are sincere and ask the question that is foremost in your mind, you will get a clear answer from the dream. If you have asked a question but your true interest lies elsewhere—or if you need to address something else within yourself before your dreaming can answer this specific question—your dream will show you that as well. Either way, do not dismiss your dream. But the next night, try to reformulate your question in view of what your dream has shown you. You can continue in this way until you get an answer.

Here is a dream from one of my students that clearly answers her question: "Am I ready to be a mother?"

> I speak with my mother, who tells me she knows she is going to die today. I feel very sad. She gives me the codes to access her accounts. There are three codes: today's date, which is the date of her death in the dream; the date of my birthday; the date of my child's birthday.

As you can see, the dream is communicative and to the point. To be reborn as a mother, the dreamer must give up being a little girl. And then after her birthday—after she is born to herself and/or after her birthday—she will conceive and have a child. The future verified her dream, as she did indeed conceive right after her birthday.

If asking your dream feels too confusing for you, or if after three weeks you have gotten no clarity, then proceed to the next exercise.

COOKING UP THE QUESTION

Do I want a child? Do I want it now? Can I afford the money or time? Is my health good enough? Does my husband want another child? How would the children feel? Am I too old or too young? Can I afford to stop working, or can I afford another child? So many questions confuse the issue. Simplifying is not easy; every aspect of the issue needs to be addressed. Is there a shortcut to the true question? Think of it as making soup. The pot is on the fire; the water is boiling. You must put many different elements into the pot to make a tasty soup. So, too, with your different questions. Put them all in the pot. Allow for time to cook. Trust the cooking. A very specific aroma will waft out of the pot when the cooking is done. Your desire to taste your soup is your bait, your question. Your dreambody's movement in response to your desire changes your body's chemistry and creates manifestation. And gives you the answer to your question.

This is what you do to make your soup:

MAKING YOUR SOUP
exercise 3

Find a quiet place in your house where you won't be disturbed. Sit in a comfortable chair, arms relaxed on the armrests, feet uncrossed, back straight. Or sit in lotus posture if you prefer. Make sure you are perfectly comfortable. Have next to you a blank notebook that you entitle *DreamBirth*. This is a different notebook from your Dream Book. In this notebook, you will record everything you sense, see, and feel in the exercises you are going to do as you follow along in this book. Choose a beautiful notebook to let your dreambody know you are serious about your intent to find out about becoming a mother. Be sure to have a pen handy.

Start the exercise at the end of your period, when you stop bleeding and your energy is no longer being pulled down. Use the upsurge of energy to question your body. You will continue the exercise until you actually hear your true question or until the start of your next period. Choose a time, morning or night—whatever suits your circumstances best. Then do not vary the time. The body forms habits and responds best to established rhythms. Read the exercise to yourself, then close your eyes.

WHAT IS MY QUESTION?
exercise 4

Close your eyes. Breathe out slowly three times, counting from 3 to 1, seeing the numbers in your mind's eye. See the number 1 as tall, clear, and bright. Ask yourself *What is my question?* Breathe out and wait to hear or see what is happening on your inner screen. If you hear or see but don't feel a strong *aha!* then breathe out and open your eyes.

Tomorrow you will repeat the exercise and repeat it again each day until you hear a clearly enunciated question and feel a strong *aha!* When you do, open your *DreamBirth* book, and on blank facing pages record exactly what you heard or saw. Do not change or alter anything.

YOUR QUESTION MADE MANIFEST

I created this exercise for myself when I had a confusion of questions such as I have outlined here. I was forty-one years old and recently married to a wonderful man who already had children. He had no desire to start another family. My doctor, my teacher, my mother, and a psychic friend independently and in the course of one month all said to me, "I think you're premenopausal." That my doctor should say so was understandable; I had symptoms. But the others? I decided I should ask my inner voice. Did I really feel the need to become a mother? I did the exercise. A week and a half into it, I heard in my native French, *"Un enfant surviendra-t-il?"* Will a child pop up unexpectedly?

I wrote the words exactly as I had heard them on a double blank page of my notebook, closed the book, and put the thought out of my mind. What I mean is, I didn't try to second-guess or obsess. My inner voice had spoken; I trusted it and went on with my business. I knew from experience that the inner voice always speaks the truth and that all I needed to do was wait for its prediction to manifest. A month later, I conceived. Because I knew the child had "popped up unexpectedly," it was easy for me to stand firm against my husband's doubts and convince him. His inner voice had long ago told him that as an older man he would have a third child. What if he had insisted, against his deeper truth, that he didn't want that child?

The inner voice speaks when we least expect it, when we are relaxed and our minds are quiet. Our inner voice is our deeper will. Against all odds, we must trust it and follow it. If we don't, we create a disruption, a separation, between our inner will and our ambitions. This makes us very unhappy. It is important to surrender to our deeper will, to accept what our depths are telling us. We must respect our deeper will, whatever the outer "sensible" course of action seems to be.

Remember that to do this exercise, your intent to know and to accept what you know must be impeccable. If you have another agenda hidden in the dark recesses of your mind, you will not get the *aha!* question that sparks manifestation. But when you do, it is imperative to follow the path that has opened up for you. You can't disrespect your inner voice without consequences.

If this tactic of asking the question fails, it means that you are not quite ready to make the commitment to your inner truth, whatever it may be. Aligning your being to your inner truth and recognizing that you are a procreator with a divine force may be your greatest test in life. Addressing your inner truth consciously and directly will open up all the other doors to creativity in your life.

I was not ready until I was forty-one to claim what I really wanted. I was always more concerned with helping others than with helping myself. So many gifts can come from asking the right question—and meeting the answers with the willingness to hear them. After I passed this major test of accepting that what I wanted was important too, and had my baby, I found out I was a poet. Poetry poured out of me: I could write! I had been mute for so many years.

THE FOUR WORLDS

As I have already said, the time to prepare for conceiving begins long before conception. It starts when the woman is still a child playing at being a mother, rehearsing her creative potential. It begins when the man is a child playing at being a father. Or maybe it begins even before that, in the unfathomable timeless depth of our subconscious.

Creation is fundamental to the human race. We are all creators. The ability to create is not limited to our physical bodies. We give birth through our various bodies: through our spiritual body inspirationally, through our mental body inventively, through our emotional body artistically, through our physical body biologically.

The process is always the same. It is described in Kabbalah as the unfolding of the four worlds.

The first world is called Atzilut, emanation. It is the initial flash, the first dot on the canvas of the universe. It is the moment when we conceive the thought of having a child or the moment when we actually conceive. It is the flash of revelation that initiates a new journey. Atzilut is often compared to the Big Bang.

The second world is called Briah, creation, where the initial flash of inspiration broadens. The first cell multiplies.

In the third world, Yetzirah, formation, plans are drawn, specific patterns begin to emerge, and cells become specialized.

In the fourth world, Assiyah, manifestation, plans become reality, patterns flesh out, babies are born.

We create our babies, our works of art, our inventions, our cities, our companies in the same unfolding way. It makes sense that for women, the act of conceiving and bringing forth babies stimulates creativity in all areas of their lives.

The more you engage the four worlds, the more creative you become. Isn't it sad to think that because we have career goals, some of us put off or deny ourselves the gift of procreating? That in our denial we limit the outpouring of creativity that is our birthright?

Think of the attention you give to a project. Without this sustained attention the project won't materialize. After your first flash of insight—Atzilut—"I'll give a surprise dinner party for my husband's birthday," you let it percolate—Briah—planning whom to invite, what kinds of food, and decorations to have. Then decisions formulate in your mind, and you make plans (Yetzirah): send out the invitations, get the decorations, buy the food. Finally it is time; all is ready to implement your plan (Assiyah): cook the meal, set the table, string up the decorations, open the door for your guests, and wait to cry, "Surprise!" when your husband walks in.

Isn't it worth giving that kind of loving attention to the conception of your child? Without it, we lose our connection to our babies, or even worse, babies die. Without proper attention, people waste away, projects fail, life withers. Do not just be the victim of nature; become a partner in creating your own destiny. Plan your conception.

PREPARING FOR CONCEPTION:
PURIFICATION OF THE FOUR BODIES

If the answer to your dream question was a resounding Yes! you have received notice from the world of Atzilut to prepare yourself for conception. If the answer comes in the form of a question, let the question permeate you. Don't try to second-guess what your still small voice is saying.

What does preparing for conception mean? As we have seen, there are four worlds and four bodies related to each. A fifth body called Yechidah is created when all four bodies work in concert. Yechidah requires loving attention, consciousness. It is the fifth force. To prepare for conception means to bring your four bodies into harmony and gathered intent—Yechidah—so as to invite a child into your life. If one of your bodies is not participating, is opposing your intent to conceive, disharmony exists even before your child's life begins. Would you plant a seed in depleted soil?

Putting all your conscious intent and loving attention into conceiving is similar to cooking a great meal. Your love activates the food and makes it tastier. How you focus and bring your emotional content to this all-important event in your life will affect your child's future, your future, and the future of all coming generations. The good food of your love will call forth a loving, peaceful child. Is this not worth your full attention?

You can prepare for conception, as we have just seen, by honing the question, or with a deliberate purification and focusing of the four bodies.

Since the four bodies are a continuum from light to dense matter— from spiritual to mental to emotional to physical—what affects one body will affect the other three. If my mental body is blocked by a belief system (i.e., *all* women in my lineage have difficult births), this will affect both my emotional and physical bodies. My emotional body will experience apprehension, anxiety, and fear. My physical body will reflect my belief system and emotional state by cramping up and following the program its other bodies inflict upon it. My spiritual body will reflect the block by shutting off hope and trust in the process of conception.

By the same token, clearing one body clears the other three. Where you start doesn't matter. You may find this hard to believe, but a change of heart can impact your physical body positively. Because imagination is the language of the body, whenever you work with images, you are affecting all the bodies. Images provoke multiple dynamic readjustments, contributing to homeostasis but also to transmutation from an obsolete state of being to a dynamic new possibility. Images move us; they are the driving agent of transformation. Remember that Yetzirah, formation, comes before Assiyah, manifestation. Wherever our life force is blocked—spiritually, mentally, emotionally, or physically—stimulating our dream flow will unblock it. Thus we can change the past, create a new future for ourselves, and activate the emergence of ever more complex states of health and well-being in the present.

CHANGING THE PAST AND CLEARING
FEARS ABOUT THE FUTURE

The past exists only inasmuch as the present contains it. Though memory may give you the illusion that it cannot be changed, your relationship to a specific memory can shift. Think of time as a curve:

you can see it from its concave or convex side, depending on where you situate yourself. Nothing, of course, prevents you from shifting places. There is a famous test, which I have reproduced here, showing a profile. Take a look at it—what do you see? Some people will see a young girl and some an old witch. Can you see both? Perception changes as we shift our eyes.

Memory is like a pop-up book. What if you could change the pop-ups? Substitute one memory for another? For example, the only memories you have of your ex-boyfriend are bad ones. But after some inner exploratory work, such as shifting your point of view to put yourself in his shoes for a moment, your anger and disappointment begin to fade. Suddenly a whole new set of memories pops up and, surprisingly, your memories now are pleasant ones. The exercises that follow will help you shift your point of view. By shifting your perception, you are allowing new possibilities to enter your consciousness.

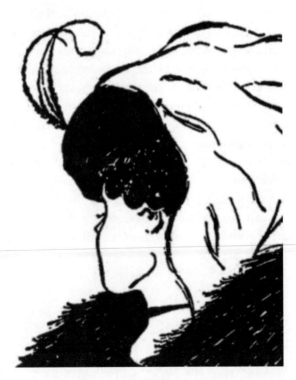

figure I   witch/young woman

Your body, which was chronically contracted because of your negative emotions, can now open up.

By disentangling your memories from painful emotions, you were able to make room for other aspects of the relationship to emerge. The energies invested in the scenes and events that constituted your memory have now been reabsorbed into the great flow of your life force. You are free to be fully present, free to energize your intentions for the future.

You no longer carry the burden of your regrets or resentments. Having absorbed the essence of your past experiences, you can turn your attention to fully enjoying your current partner and together, with an open heart, begin to prepare for the conception of your child.

To clear the resentments of the past and the fears about the future, we will address four areas: 1) old relationships that still cling to you; 2) abortions and miscarriages; 3) blocked emotions; 4) personal and ancestral belief systems. I've chosen to focus on these four because these are the areas where most women get bogged down.

MOVING PAST OLD RELATIONSHIPS

Today most of us experience more than one sexual partner before settling down to a committed relationship. Those experiences affect us, whether we like it or not. We exchange in more than just physical ways. Mingling our emotional and subtle bodies with those of others cannot be done with impunity. Memories, images, fears, regrets, resentments, and anger may linger. If you are still dreaming of your first lover or ranting against the man who left you for your best friend, you need to clear away the emotions caught in the fabric of your memories. Your dreams, fantasies, and behaviors tell you when you are still attached to an old flame, and your attachment can be in desiring that person or in holding a lot of anger or hatred toward that person. You may have the very best relationship with your new partner, be madly in love and deeply committed, but this does not automatically clear the past. To do so, you need to become proactive: to find a quicker way to clear out unwanted residue from past relationships than dissecting and analyzing every difficult event of your history. Here is a simple exercise to help you do that.

EMPTYING YOUR HANDBAG
exercise 5

Close your eyes. Breathe out slowly three times, counting from
3 to 1, seeing the numbers in your mind's eye. See the number
1 as tall, clear, and bright.

You're at the beach. It's a bright, sunny day. The sky is blue.
See the ocean as calm and very blue, with mild waves.

Breathe out. Take off your shoes and socks, roll up your pant legs,
and step into the ocean up to your knees, holding your handbag.

Breathe out. Open your handbag. Throw into the ocean
anything in your handbag that is not absolutely necessary for
your survival.

Breathe out. See how the waves are sweeping these objects
away and into the depths of the ocean.

Breathe out. What do you throw out and what do you keep?

Breathe out. Turn your bag inside out and wash it in the ocean.
Then put it out to dry in the sun.

Breathe out. When the bag is dry, turn it outside in and put in
the few objects you are keeping, if any.

Breathe out. Holding your bag, walk away, feeling lighter
and freer.

Breathe out. Open your eyes.

Your womb is like your handbag, a receptacle for old and new attachments. It is in your womb that you store memories of empowerment and joy or trauma affecting your ability to create. I remember once passing my hands over a student and seeing, in my mind's eye, a rabbit in her womb and a sobbing six-year-old. When I told her, she burst into tears: "My daddy killed my rabbit when I was six years old!" Although we cleared the memory, the habit of fear in her body was too great. She was not able to conceive, but she was able to become a mother. She adopted a wonderful little girl.

Memories are in your cells, located in different parts of your body. It is in your womb that you store your memories of lovers who have participated with you in the sexual dance. These images and strata of experiences are very real to your physical body.

But now you are in another phase of your life. You need to clear the old memories that do not serve you. Think of it as clearing your closet of old clothes. Memories also take up space you need to free up and allow new things to happen.

To be sure that you have liberated yourself completely from past specific relationships, do this exercise.

CLEARING YOUR WOMB
exercise 6

Close your eyes. Breathe out slowly three times, counting from 3 to 1, seeing the numbers in your mind's eye. See the number 1 as tall, clear, and bright.

Turning your eyes inward, let your gaze travel down into your womb. See all the cords that still attach you to former partners.

Breathe out. Identifying each cord with a former partner, thank the man for what he has taught you, then firmly cut the cord that still attaches you to him, knowing that you are returning his energy to him and, in the process, restoring your own completeness.

Breathe out. Continue doing this for each cord until all are cut.

Breathe out. Pour fresh spring water into your womb. See your womb as clean and bright.

Breathe out. Feel refreshed and restored to wholeness, ready to receive your partner of choice, the one your heart has singled out to be the father of your child.

Breathe out. Open your eyes.

Clearing old relationships that still resonate also requires that you take some practical actions, such as cleaning your closets and bedroom. Do you still cling to nostalgic remnants of days gone by, objects that are no longer relevant to your present life and new intentions? Throwing them away is usually a good idea, but if you like to keep mementos, keep only those that bring a smile to your face. Clothes, mattresses, curtains hold the old energies. Objects store memories. If throwing things away is not practical, or even if it is, cleaning your bedroom is essential. While the following exercise is done purely in your imagination, get into the habit, whenever you physically clean your bedroom or take a shower, of intending to clean your interior at the same time. This works very well.

CLEANING YOUR BEDROOM
exercise 7

Close your eyes. Breathe out slowly three times, counting from 3 to 1, seeing the numbers in your mind's eye. See the number 1 as tall, clear, and bright.

Imagine you are gathering your supplies—broom, sponge, duster, pail of soapy water—to clean your bedroom.

Breathe out. Begin to clean, sensing every movement of your body as you scrub the ceiling, the walls, from top to bottom, the windows inside and out.

Breathe out. Open closets and chests of drawers, putting everything you no longer need or find useful into a large black garbage bag. Dust and clean the closets and drawers.

Breathe out. Take the rugs to the window and beat the dust out of them.

Breathe out. Move the furniture. Turn the mattress over. Wash the floor.

Breathe out. When you have finished cleaning your room, rearrange the furniture.

Breathe out. Now place what you mean to keep in closets and drawers. Make your bed with clean, new sheets.

Breathe out. Take all your supplies and wash or clean them before putting them away.

Breathe out. Carry the black garbage bag out to a garbage truck, throw it into the truck, and watch as it is crushed. Then watch the truck drive away.

Breathe out. When you have completely cleared and rearranged your bedroom to your satisfaction, find and bring into your room a special object or flower arrangement that gives you pleasure and enhances the room.

Breathe out. Open your eyes, seeing your clean new bedroom with open eyes.

This exercise may be more powerful than you think. I remember giving it to a young woman who was having repetitive dreams of a young man leaning out of a castle bedroom window on a full moonlit night while, beyond the castle walls, she looked longingly up at this unattainable prince. The day after I had her do the exercise, she called me in a frenzy of grief and repentance. She confessed she was earning her living as a call girl. The imagined cleaning of her bedroom had provoked the change she dreaded and most longed for. She gave up being a call girl and found a more "soul" appropriate way of making her living.

Images, because they are experienced with all their accompanying sensations, can effect profound and often instantaneous transformations in our lives.

ABORTIONS: REPAIRING THE IRREPARABLE

As I have noted, the physical body lives subconsciously, carrying in its cells many memories that only surface when dislodged by outside circumstances. Thoughts of having a child can bring these submerged memories to consciousness, awakening old grievances, pain, and confusion.

An unwanted pregnancy terminated by an abortion can leave just such painful traces in our cells. Regardless of the fact that many women are pro-choice politically, deep down, a woman most often will experience abortion as a violation of her life force and that of her unborn child. Women who have had abortions, however justified by circumstances—a result of financial circumstances, teenage pregnancy, the wrong partner, a one-night stand, rape, or health considerations—may still be carrying around a heavy burden of guilt. One student who had an abortion and later had difficulty conceiving saw images of her right ovary as a bright light and her left ovary covered by a shadow. She had a hard time sweeping the shadow away. When I asked her to address the shadow, it turned out to be the little boy she had aborted. This next exercise will allow you to meet the soul you didn't get to meet. It will alleviate your sadness and reassure you that your potential child is doing all right.

CLEANING OUT AN ABORTION
exercise 8

Close your eyes. Breathe out slowly three times, counting from 3 to 1, seeing the numbers in your mind's eye. See the number 1 as tall, clear, and bright.

Call on the soul of your lost child. You can see it appearing as a pair of little red shoes. Ask your child to forgive you, explaining to her the reasons for your actions (e.g., you couldn't support the child, you weren't married, you were selfish, you were too young, or your parents would be angry). Give all the reasons.

Breathe out. Hear what the child says. If the child won't forgive you, ask what she needs you to do or promise her in order for her to forgive.

Breathe out. Once you have made an agreement (life affirming for you and acceptable to her), thank the child for her forgiveness and promise her that from now on, you will respect life.

Breathe out. Ask the child if she intends to come back to you. Tell the child now is a time when you can receive her safely. Hear what she says.

Breathe out. Say good-bye to your child and see the little red shoes moving away and disappearing.

Breathe out. Open your eyes, feeling absolved and open to the future.

When a woman feels free of guilt, her body relaxes and conception is more likely to happen. Taking care of unfinished business allows your body to bloom again. The relief and lightness that come from making peace with the child you had to abandon allows you to look forward to the future with hope and anticipation. Your anticipation will be all the sweeter if the child has told you she will come back.

CLEARING BLOCKED EMOTIONS

What if instead of the past, you fear the future? You have had a couple of miscarriages and fear having another, or your doctor has spoken of congenital malformation of the embryo, and you fear having a disabled child. Or, having seen how your parents behaved toward their children, you fear that you may behave like them when you become a parent. Fear, worry, and anxiety affect both your ability to conceive and the quality of your consciousness at the time of conception. Just as any emotional shock can affect your pregnancy, the same is true as your body prepares to create. The time before conception is as important for the future of your child as is your time of pregnancy.

Fears about the future are almost always based on the past and on the false assumption that the past will repeat itself in the future. How does one assuage the fears of a woman who has had a couple of miscarriages? The fearful anticipation of just such an event could shut down her various bodies. Fear does a good job of convincing us that our worries are legitimate. If you adopt fear, you will find it so powerful that it will manifest what you most dread. If, on the other hand, you believe that mind comes before matter and not the other way around, it is possible to shift out of fear and embody a completely different point of view. Fear will always try to convince you that you are wrong. You must find the courage and determination to move away from fear toward the miraculous and the unknown. It takes great audacity to endorse the idea that an unknown good awaits you in the future. Choose audacity.

TO GET RID OF FEAR
exercise 9

Close your eyes. Breathe out slowly three times, counting from 3 to 1, seeing the numbers in your mind's eye. See the number 1 as tall, clear, and bright.

See yourself in a meadow on a bright, sunny day. Reach your hands up toward the sun. When your hands are close to the sun, sense them becoming very warm and turning into light.

Breathe out. Now bring your hands into your body, gather up all your fears, take them out of your body, and throw them up into the heavens. Watch as the heavens dissolve them.

Breathe out. Open your eyes.

As I have said, getting rid of your fears is not sufficient. If you don't replace them with something else, they will return. Dare to believe in a miracle. You don't know what that miracle will be, but trusting makes all the difference. Trusting is the attitude of the wise virgins in the parable of the bridegroom.[12] They are called virgins because they have pushed away fear; they hold in their cupped hands the lamp and oil that light their way. They remain awake to possibility. "Therefore, stay awake, for you know neither the day nor the hour." Like the wise virgins, believe in the great flow of life and abundance. This is a loving attitude. Whereas fear constricts, love radiates out like a star. You cannot constrict when you are expanded. It is physically impossible.

MANNA FROM HEAVEN
exercise 10

Close your eyes. Breathe out slowly three times, counting from 3 to 1, seeing the numbers in your mind's eye. See the number 1 as tall, clear, and bright.

Having thrown your fears up to the heavens, hold your cupped hands open to receive the manna of heaven. Watch what comes into your hands.

Breathe out. Be grateful for what you receive.

Breathe out. Open your eyes.

Expansion is what allows life into you. You can hold yourself ready for whatever will come from heaven and trust that it will be for your highest good.

PERSONAL AND ANCESTRAL BELIEF SYSTEMS

Our belief systems are so familiar to us that we don't even know we have them. They are insidious that way. They can only be dislodged by a major confrontation or cataclysm. I remember a very bright and liberal friend of mine telling me that as a child he sat in the seats reserved for whites in the South's segregated buses and never once thought to question their injustice until Rosa Parks made her historic statement on behalf of all blacks.

While there are great and small belief systems, all of them affect us, blocking our ability to see life from a different point of view or to act differently. You may have heard your grandmother say that you had narrow hips and would have difficulty giving birth as a result. Your mother, catching you touching yourself, said no man would ever marry you. You heard a friend telling your father your smile would damn a saint, and you decided never to smile again. The thought enters your brain unquestioned and lodges there like a mole, programming you to fulfill its prediction. The only way you can become aware that something is wrong is by paying attention to your repetitive patterns of behavior and thought.

IDENTIFYING REPETITIVE BEHAVIORS OR THOUGHTS
exercise II

Close your eyes. Breathe out slowly three times, counting from 3 to 1, seeing the numbers in your mind's eye. See the number 1 as tall, clear, and bright.

Look back on your life and identify a repetitive behavior or thought.

Breathe out. Once you have identified it, ask to be shown the source of the behavior or thought you have been repeating.

Breathe out. If the source is a person, imagine going into your brain and finding the tape of that person's message. Take it out of your brain and return it to the person, saying, "I return to Caesar what belongs to Caesar." Make sure that person takes the tape from you.

Breathe out. If it is not a person but a thought you had, see the thought in front of you, then stretch your hand up to catch a ray of the sun. Use it as a laser to dissolve the thought into light.

Breathe out. Pour spring water where the tape or thought was lodged in your brain and ask every cell in your body to return to its natural, healthy alignment.

Breathe out. Open your eyes.

More insidious still are family patterns. French psychologists have studied this strange phenomenon of repetitive behaviors within family lines. For instance, the great grandfather, grandfather, and father, unbeknownst to their wives and family, each had a secret mistress. While their behavior remains unknown to the son, he engages in the same double life as his father, grandfather, and great grandfather. Stranger still, the women in a lineage may all die around the same age from car crashes. The outside world seems to conspire with the subconscious family patterns. What is really happening? Once a belief system is programmed into your subconscious, it acts like a repetitive dream. Unless you clear it out of your subconscious, it will continue like a broken record to program your body to act a certain way. Dream patterns are shared by all those connected to your dreamfield. Family members are the most prone to picking up on them.

CLEARING ANCESTRAL BELIEFS ABOUT CONCEPTION
exercise 12

Close your eyes. Breathe out slowly three times, counting from 3 to 1, seeing the numbers in your mind's eye. See the number 1 as tall, clear, and bright.

Imagine that you are in the house of your ancestors. Climb up to the attic, look around, and find the old chest that you have been told contains your family's ancestral beliefs about conception and childbirth.

Breathe out. Open the chest. What do you find?

Breathe out. Keep what you like and discard the rest. Make a pile of what you are discarding and take it out to the garden to burn. Then bury the ashes.

Breathe out. Walk away with what you have kept.

Breathe out. Open your eyes.

CHANGING YOUR FAMILY HISTORY

In the 1950s it was believed that women should be drugged when giving birth. Tomorrow, it may be considered uncivilized to carry your child in your own womb, and you will hire a surrogate, just as in the Middle Ages when women of high society hired a wet nurse to suckle their babies. It takes a rebel or a revolution to change patterns of thought or behavior, and the best rebel is the dreamer. As a dreamer you are not fixed in one position; you can easily change yours. All you have to do is imagine that you are standing in another location or in another's shoes. From that new vantage point, you will see things differently. You may see something you had never seen before. Suddenly you are thinking differently.

A TAPESTRY OF YOUR FAMILY HISTORY
exercise 13

Close your eyes. Breathe out slowly three times, counting from 3 to 1, seeing the numbers in your mind's eye. See the number 1 as tall, clear, and bright.

See yourself at your loom weaving a tapestry of your family history. As you weave, see your entire ancestral history even if you don't know everything about it.

Breathe out. Weave the history of your ancestors back and forth all day long until, at nightfall, you finish the tapestry. Experience all the sensations, emotions, pains, and pleasures that come with the completion of the tapestry.

Breathe out. At nightfall, start undoing the tapestry. Undo it until you have taken it completely apart. Pay attention to your sensations and emotions. Be aware that as you undo your tapestry, you are clearing away everything that needs to be cleared away in your family. Do this until daybreak.

Breathe out. As the first rays of the sun appear, weave a new tapestry containing only the good and new possibilities your ancestral line carries. Weave into your tapestry all the good and powerful qualities your line has developed throughout its many generations and all the new potential it carries—to inform, instruct, and support you in a future that is filled with joy, health, and success.

Breathe out. See yourself now weaving into your tapestry the story of your child being gestated perfectly, born perfectly, and growing perfectly into its future.

Breathe out. Open your eyes, seeing your magnificent new creation.

Having cleared the past of your worries about the future to the best of your abilities, you are ready for your bodies to begin the great pilgrimage of unfolding into their new intent: inviting a child into your womb. You have packed lightly, discarding what you don't need on your journey. Your next move is setting out on the journey.

Your active dreaming has shown you that you can affect your attitudes toward the past. You have discarded old belief systems and stagnant emotions. You may be feeling a little lost without these old crutches; the way forward is unknown. But you are undertaking this journey with a clear intent. You have begun to verify that the process works. Keep verifying as you step lightly into your life with hopes high and a smile in your heart. Remember: the best dreamer is the one who dares to go with the changes her images offer up to her. Trust your dreaming to show you the way.

2

CONCEPTION

Calling Forth a Soul

For this reason a man shall leave his father and mother and be
joined to his wife, and the two shall become one flesh.

GENESIS 2:24

THE OLD TEACHINGS say that it takes three to make a child: father, mother, and the Divine. In the last chapter, we discussed the mother and the Divine. What about the father? He is the mirror image of his female counterpart. While her body is soft, his is firm; while her sexual organs are turned inward, his are turned outward; while she has bosoms, his breasts are flat. They fit into each other as two pieces of a puzzle. In the old myths, he and she were once one, but then they were parted, desire awoke (even if the partners are of the same biological sex, their energy bodies will be either male or female, which explains their desire for each other). Desire is the longing, fueled by the vision, to be united and become one again. But we live in linear time. We can only manifest our lost unity through a child.

Everything in this world is in relationship; nothing exists on its own. Your desire expresses itself through your senses. The old teachings say that if you focus on what you desire, holding that image steadily in your mind and feeling it strongly in your heart, you will manifest what you desire. This is why it is so important to clear and steady your mind, to know what your true desire is. Think of it as heart-mind technology. The best-selling book *The Secret* has made this technology popular, but there is a very big catch. If your desire-image—of yourself as a successful provider, for example—is masking a deeper belief system that you will always be a failure, your subconscious (the language of your body) has no choice but to follow the orders implicit in the images containing that deeper belief system. No matter how hard you visualize being successful, if you haven't cleared those failure images and their damaging emotions, you will not be able to gain success. It would be like slapping a cheerful poster onto a rotting wall. It won't stop the rot from continuing its insidious work. So be sure to take a moment to know yourself and to check for what you really want.

Be careful what you wish for. Be very specific in concentrating on the good qualities you see in your partner and yourself or in the family members and ancestors you admire. Your desire-image, once purified

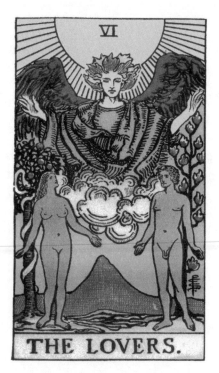

figure 2   tarot lover's card

of false belief systems, acts like an arrow. What you see and love in each other (and in your families through each other) is what you will manifest. How you focus your desire determines the outcome. Both of you are important in this equation and need to play your parts. You must match each other in the power of your desire and focus. In the card depicting the Lovers from the tarot deck, the man is looking at the woman, who is gazing up at a resplendent angel. The angel is said to be Archangel Raphael, one of the seven holy angels that attend the throne of God. He is the angel of healing. Does something need to be healed between the lovers?

Clearly, the card depicts something to do with the relationship between the man and the woman. In the Devil card, which is uncannily similar in layout to the Lovers card but opposite in meaning, the man and woman are not free but bound by chains to a half-cube, upon which sits the Devil, winged in parody of the angel. He is

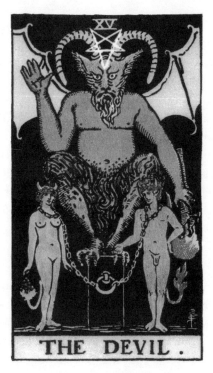

figure 3   devil tarot card

igniting the tail of the man who looks pointedly at the woman's sex. Her body is turned toward his, but her face looks away. They are at cross-purposes. Sexuality for the sake of one's own selfish pleasure keeps both partners in bondage. Yet the chains around the necks of the man and woman are loose and easy to slip out of. All it requires is a shift from selfish appetites to purified desire.

Would you not want your images to look as much as possible like your higher selves, like the incorruptible image of the Divine in you, to which the archangel in the Lovers card is alluding? Your child's future well-being depends on what you are envisioning as you come together. The range of possibilities from bestiality to angelic humanity is huge. If you believe, as I do, that mind comes before matter, it is your responsibility to purify your mind as you begin your journey toward a conscious conception.

PREPARING FOR CONCEPTION

Parenting begins before conception. As parents, you will soon learn that mixed signals create confusion and disorder. You must agree on how you are going to bring up your child. It is best to have a vision you both share, one that conforms to your higher desire for happiness and harmonious growth. You will want to be "in sync" with each other.

As I write, I am counseling a young couple, who love each other deeply and are committed to having children together. The young wife is the woman who dreamed that, at the time of her birthday, she would be ready to conceive. After she told her husband, he dreamed he wasn't quite ready yet. He had many work obligations that would take him traveling, and he wanted her to be able to travel with him. She was very hurt. How could work be more important than having a child? He was clear he would be ready in a few months, but she was ready now, and she felt sure the child was ready too. What if delaying would spoil their chances of conceiving? He felt she was pushing him and resented it. In a case like this, trying to determine who is right will only make matters worse. How to respect each other's rhythms and needs when these conflicts arise is the question. Logic cannot solve the issue.

When emotions are very raw, it is best at first not to try to thrash it out but instead to step back for a while.

TAKE THREE STEPS BACK
exercise 14

Close your eyes. Breathe out slowly three times, counting from 3 to 1, seeing the numbers in your mind's eye. See the number 1 as tall, clear, and bright.

Imagine that you take three steps back, sensing your movements. Breathe out. Now look at your partner—what do you feel?

(If there is no change either in the way you see your partner or in your feelings toward your partner, take three more steps back. You can do this three times if needed.)

Breathe out. Open your eyes.

If you still disagree about the timing of conception, you may not be ready to discuss the issue calmly after doing this exercise, but you can communicate "through the airways." What does that mean? I'm sure you've noticed how you can often pick up, before it is verbalized, what another person is thinking. You can also pick up the other's moods, emotions, and sensations. Through your emotional involvement, you are attuned to your partner, just as you tune in to your favorite TV station by clicking on the right channel. You are able to pick up on your nonverbal right-brain screen what the other is experiencing in the form of images. Being attuned emotionally means that you move in interwoven frequency fields. This is why husbands and wives often dream similar dreams at night; dreaming is contagious. You can use the permeability of dreaming to send images of love or reparation. Images speak louder than words about your desire for reconciliation. To bring about a restored harmony, do this next exercise.

RETURN TO A PLACE OF LOVE
exercise 15

Close your eyes. Breathe out slowly three times, counting from 3 to 1, seeing the numbers in your mind's eye. See the number 1 as tall, clear, and bright.

Imagine retiring to your bedroom or to a place of harmony, like a garden or meadow, where you can feel quiet.

Breathe out. Return to the first time you fell in love with your current partner. See the moment and feel it. What color is the love in your heart?

Breathe out. Send this color as a bridge of light from your heart to your partner's heart. Whatever you want to say or show, send it over the bridge of light to your partner.

Breathe out. Listen and watch. You may receive a message in return.

Breathe out. Feeling more at peace, open your eyes.

You will find that it is easier to communicate through your dreaming. Friction diminishes because the story you have settled on in your mind is less in evidence. Dreaming is the language of the subconscious, and it will lead you by ways that are less logical but more "knowing." This is easy since, as I have said, you are naturally attuned to each other through your emotions.

40

HARMONIZING TOGETHER

We are each of us a world unto ourselves. We swim in a vast universe of memories, emotions, narratives, and sensations. That we can harmonize with one another is nothing short of miraculous. "The heart has its reasons that reason knows not."[13] When the harmony is there, we are filled with joy; we dance together in a symphony of rhythms. We are in love. But we live in a world of limitations, and our dance is inevitably interrupted. We first register disharmony in our own body rhythms. Our breath, our heartbeats, and our movements become uneven. We must work to restore harmony. Becoming conscious of our own rhythms and then becoming responsible for them are both simple.

NATURAL BREATHING
exercise 16

Close your eyes. Bring your attention down into your body.

Watch your breathing without trying to change it . . . allowing it to find its natural rhythm . . . knowing that when it returns to its natural rhythm, what is not in place tends to return to be in place.

Breathe out. Open your eyes.

When you have learned to pay attention to your own breathing, you will notice more easily how the presence of certain people or situations affects your breathing. Your body is always assessing outer stress and seeking balance through what is called homeostasis. Your changed rhythms alert you to potential danger. Your emotions—manifesting through those changed movements in your body—tell you what you are feeling about the other. You have been given a wonderful tool to help you in your evolution, and you need to pay attention to it. If you collapse into the emotion, you will not be able to be present to what is happening within you. Identifying the emotion will help you to communicate with your partner. It is a simple matter of saying, "When you act this way or speak to me this way, this is what I feel." Your partner will not be able to contradict you, since it is your feeling. Respecting what each other feels without trying to solve the problem is your best way into deeper knowing. This place of nonjudgment will help both of you come to a resolution that matches your individual needs. To help with reestablishing harmony, do the simple exercise that follows.

REPOTTING THE PLANT
exercise 17

Close your eyes. Breathe out slowly three times, counting from 3 to 1, seeing the numbers in your mind's eye. See the number 1 as tall, clear, and bright.

Imagine a potted plant in your home that isn't doing well.

Breathe out. Decide to break the pot in which it sits. Free the roots of the plant from the old soil.

Breathe out. Gather all the pieces of the old pot and the old soil into a black garbage bag. Take the garbage bag out and throw it into a garbage truck that is driving by.

Breathe out. You have prepared a bigger and more beautiful new pot for your plant. Fill it with fresh, rich, dark soil.

Breathe out. Plant your plant in the rich, new soil.

Breathe out. Take a pitcher of clear spring water and water your plant. Watch what happens.

Breathe out. Open your eyes.

You will feel well together if you are sharing rhythms. Your bodies are your unique musical instruments. Start with the simplest of rhythms, your breaths. To perfectly harmonize as a couple, practice together or separately the harmonizing breath.

HARMONIZING BREATH
exercise 18

Close your eyes. Breathe out slowly three times, counting from 3 to 1, seeing the numbers in your mind's eye. See the number 1 as tall, clear, and bright.

See yourself in front of your partner. Pay attention to the rhythm of his breathing. Now watch the rhythm of your own breathing.

What is the difference between these two rhythms?

Breathe out. Imagine that a pendulum swings, from left to right and right to left, in the space between you. Feel how the pendulum is finding an in-between rhythm. What happens to your breathing and to the breathing of your partner? How do you feel now?

Breathe out. Open your eyes.

Being attuned is not a fixed state but a constantly changing land-scape. Think of it as musical improvisation. The better able you are to improvise counterpoint to the *cantus firmus,* or fixed song of your partnership, the better attuned you will be to each other. This attunement is an art that is crucial to your ability to be in a vibrant relationship. The more you refine your art, the more apt you are to come to a peak moment of harmonization when you decide to con-ceive. Being in harmony at the moment of conceiving assures that your child's initial Big Bang into this world is at its optimum best.

CONCEIVING CONSCIOUSLY

Where do we come from, and where are we going? Are we immortals incarnating into this world and, after living our life span, departing to subtler realms? Or are we simply genetic accidents that appear and disap-pear, "dust to dust and ashes to ashes," leaving no traces? It is important to spend a moment reflecting on these mysteries, as your answers will kindle the humility you need to approach this awesome moment of creat-ing a new life. Whatever your answer to yourself is, the mystery of where your child comes from remains profound. Life's source is always a mystery.

GRATITUDE (1)
exercise 19

Close your eyes. Breathe out slowly three times, counting from 3 to 1, seeing the numbers in your mind's eye. See the number 1 as tall, clear, and bright.

Sense, see, and feel where you come from. How have you been true or untrue to your origins? Repair what you need to repair.

Breathe out. Sense, see, and feel where your potential child comes from. What are your belief systems surrounding the mystery of conception?

Breathe out. Sense and feel the mystery.

Breathe out. See and feel that your child is a gift from sovereign life to your life. When you have seen, feel all the gratitude that a gift brings with it.

Breathe out. Open your eyes, feeling the gratitude.

If you have looked into the vast pool of mystery in the eyes of newborns, or if you have heard your children calling long before they were conceived, you can make sense of the preexistence of the soul in a celestial world. Whether you relate to your future child as a preexisting soul or as your higher self, when you imagine your future child, you need to ask—as you would when anticipating the arrival of a very special guest—what your guest's special needs and requests might be.

TO CALL FORTH A SOUL
exercise 20

Close your eyes. Breathe out slowly three times, counting from 3 to 1, seeing the numbers in your mind's eye. See the number 1 as tall, clear, and bright.

Imagine that you are standing in a meadow looking up at the sky on a clear day. See a white cloud floating gently out from the left side of the blue sky and see the soul of your child appearing on this cloud.

Breathe out. When your child appears, ask him what you need to do to prepare for his arrival. What changes must you make in your physical, emotional, and mental bodies for your child to be able to incarnate? Pay great attention to the answer.

Breathe out. When you have heard and seen, promise your child to promptly do what is necessary to secure his arrival. Thank him for being patient.

Breathe out. Open your eyes.

You must not only align yourself with your coming child but with the natural laws that govern the world you live in, for these are the pathways and portals through which your child travels to reach you. The ways in which the cycles, rotations, and movements of the planets and stars in the galaxy interact with your own particular chart has something to say about when your child can be conceived. The waxing and waning of the moon in particular, in conjunction with your birth dates and those of your family, plays an important role in when you can actually conceive.

When is the right time to conceive? It has been scientifically established that a woman's ovulation is her time of greatest fertility, and this was known to ancient people many thousands of years ago. Jewish marriages, for instance, are timed to coincide with the woman's ovulation, for the first sexual encounter of a couple is expected to be filled with the most intense desire and love and is therefore thought propitious for conceiving. But what you do not know is that family birth dates play an important role in when, during those times of ovulation, you are most likely to conceive. You will exhaust yourself if you do not follow the laws of nature.

The following system was developed by Colette Aboulker-Muscat and has served us well in determining the most propitious times for conception. Having paid attention for many years to the family birth dates registered at the Algiers Hospital where she worked, Colette observed that there were specific and recurring birth patterns in families.

FINDING THE MOST PROPITIOUS
DATES FOR CONCEIVING
exercise 21

Make a list of the family birth dates—day and month (the year is not important)—of your siblings, parents, grandparents, and great grandparents. Go back as far as you can. Observe the recurring dates. Start first by observing how many times the same month appears. Within that month, what are the recurring dates? Your window of opportunity lies within three days before and after the common dates. Once the dates are established, calculate every three months from your original date. Those resonant times are also propitious.

For example:

	Mother's line	Father's line
Parents	November 1	February 8
	May 1	March 27
Siblings	May 20	October 30
	July 28	
Children of siblings	April 13	October 1
		July 22
Mother (yourself)	December 12	Father July 6
Existing child	February 28	

Possible dates of conception—calculated to your nearest ovulation time—are going to be the end of October, the beginning of November, the end of July, and the end of February.

1) July 25—October 25—January 25—April 25—July 25
2) November 1—February 1—May 1—August 1—November 1
3) February 28—May 28—August 28—November 28—February 28

So if your ovulation peak is July 30, that will be your potential conception date for July.

This simple method works. You can calculate it yourself and easily verify its accuracy by checking whether you, your siblings, and your partner were indeed conceived during family birth dates or resonant times.

For more complex calculations and fertility times that are outside the ovulation period, look up the Jonas method, developed in the 1950s by a Slovakian doctor, Dr. Eugen Jonas. He discovered that in addition to their regular fertility cycle, women have another cycle, which he called the Lunar Fertility Cycle. Dr. Jonas uses the relative positions of the sun and the moon at the moment of a woman's birth to determine the best moments for conception. This method has received widespread recognition and claims a 97-percent accuracy rate for conception and 85 percent for gender selection. To use it, you will need to know your birth date and the hour at which you were born.

Having chosen the dates, your last action must be to prepare the space in which to receive your guest. This is akin to creating a perfect space to house your most precious jewel. Make it beautiful in the physical realm so that every sense is enhanced. On the inner plane, use your intent and your joy to create the sacred space and make it irresistible.

SHINING YOUR OVARIES AND UTERUS
exercise 22

Close your eyes. Breathe out slowly three times, counting from 3 to 1, seeing the numbers in your mind's eye. See the number 1 as tall, clear, and bright.

Imagine that you are standing in a meadow on a clear, sunny day. Look up at the sun. Stretch your arms toward the sun, feel them getting longer and longer. Feel your hands getting warm, your fingers turning into light. See a little hand appearing at the tip of each finger. Now you have fifty little fingers of light.

Breathe out. Bring your fifty little fingers down into your body to illuminate your ovaries.

Breathe out. Start massaging one of your ovaries with your fifty little fingers of light until your ovary becomes as bright and shining as a star.

Breathe out. Massage the other ovary until it, too, is as bright and shining as a star.

Breathe out. Lift your hands up toward the sun again. Feel the little hands disappearing back into your fingers. Gather a bouquet of sun rays. Bring it down to you as your arms return to their normal length.

Breathe out. Roll the sun rays into a perfect ball of sunlight. Put it into your uterus. See it rolling around the inside of your uterus, clearing whatever needs to be cleared and coating it with golden oil.

Breathe out. Return the ball of sunlight to the sun.

Breathe out. Open your eyes, seeing your two starry ovaries and the sun of your uterus with open eyes.

You are now ready to carry forth your intentions. Your inner and outer houses are ready. Encourage your partner to do his own work (see chapter 8 for DreamBirth exercises your partner can do). Your two beings are attuned to carry forth your intention and perform the magical act of creation, which makes you partners with the Divine. Your full participation is called for.

CONCEPTION

Folk wisdom is clear: it is not good to conceive in anger, fear, sadness, resentment, or against one's will. It is not good to come together while fantasizing about another. In fact, kabbalists believe that the intent during sexual union has the power to bring "good" to the world. Lack of inward intent or distraction can cause major disruptions in the order and coherence of the universe. Kabbalists and Buddhists alike believe that when two people make love, they create a "spirit body" into which the soul pours itself. Kabbalists call this creating a *diyok'na,* a spirit image that is the garment of the soul. Keeping your love intent strong, clear, and focused on the higher good, the spirit form to which you both aspire, is crucial.

The exercise you are about to do is very ancient and was given by kabbalists to women to help them conceive. Do not read it unless you are ready to sit down and do it. Do it only once.

❦

THE CONCEPTION EXERCISE
exercise 23

Close your eyes. Breathe out slowly three times, counting from 3 to 1, seeing the numbers in your mind's eye. See the number 1 as tall, clear, and bright.

Imagine that you are looking up at an emerald-green hill at the summit of which is a magnificent tree. Describe the tree to yourself.

Breathe out. As you start walking up the hill, see your partner coming up the other side of the hill.

Breathe out. Feel the loving and intense desire to meet. As you reach each other, embrace, hold hands, and sit under the tree.

Breathe out. See the blue dome of the sky descending to envelop the tree and both of you.

Breathe out. See that a spark of blue light detaches itself from inside the dome, enters your womb, and attaches itself there.

Breathe out. See this bright light in your womb.

Breathe out. The dome of the sky returns to its place in the firmament. The light glows in your womb.

Breathe out. Get up and walk hand in hand down the hill, seeing the glowing light in your womb.

Breathe out. Open your eyes.

You have met imaginally and conceived from the light. Now you must also meet physically. Following is an exercise to enhance your desire and love for each other. You can use it whenever you want to meet physically or simply to stimulate your passion for each other. It is written from the woman's point of view, but it also can be done from the man's point of view. Just notice that orange is for the woman and red for the man.

MEADOW COLORS
exercise 24

Close your eyes. Breathe out slowly three times, counting from 3 to 1, seeing the numbers in your mind's eye. See the number 1 as tall, clear, and bright.

See that you are in a large, very lush green meadow. On the other side of the meadow, see your partner. Feel excited and happy to see him.

Breathe out. As you walk toward each other, see what color he emanates, what color you emanate.

Breathe out. See the colors getting more and more vibrant and warmer. See him becoming a brighter and brighter red and see yourself becoming more and more brightly orange.

Breathe out. When you meet and the two colors come together, see what is created.

Breathe out. Open your eyes, seeing what is created with open eyes.

Both of you can practice this exercise as many times as you want. If you know that you are ready to conceive, practice it every night before going to bed. Remember that by focusing on each other to the exclusion of all else except the mystery that unites you, you enhance the power of your creation. The greatest power of all is love, but we are often distracted from love by the pull of our daily obligations. It is good to set the stage, to prepare the space for enhanced joy and harmony. If you meditate and have an altar, you have probably spent time ornamenting your altar—placing a flower on it, burning incense, lighting a candle—to invite your guest in. This is the same as that. You will wish to invite each other into the sacred space where you come together to create. You may want to bring to each other something special that speaks of your love for each other. A gift adds joy and appreciation. Then, together, sit face to face and do this next exercise.

TWO MIRRORS
exercise 25

Close your eyes. Breathe out slowly three times, counting from 3 to 1, seeing the numbers in your mind's eye. See the number 1 as tall, clear, and bright.

See the two of you as two mirrors reflecting each other in the eloquent silence that is eternity.

Breathe out. At this place of inner vision, we shall see the place where I and Thou do not exist.

Breathe out. Know that it is only by words of silence that love becomes complete. Hear this garland of silent words and enjoy the perfect meeting.

Breathe out. Open your eyes, feeling the perfect meeting with open eyes.

Remember that, like the faithful virgins in the parable told by Jesus Christ,[14] you may have to wait for your guest to arrive. Your time of waiting can seem very long. You may have unrequited hopes and setbacks that affect you. Do not despair. Know that waiting is one of the great tools for transformation, used by many religious disciplines to develop inner strength and intent. Continue to prepare. By gathering your energy, you are building up a great storage of power. Use it to come together with ever-mounting love and faith. You are learning courage, the power of the heart to attract to you "a holy soul."

When your child finally makes his entry into your lives, you will know that he is the one you were meant to host, the one you called forth together with all your heart, with all your soul, and with all your strength.

PART TWO

Milestones of Pregnancy

3

Exciting News

I've put seeds in the ground and I'm waiting for an answer.

BEDOUIN IN THE NEGEV

A NEW WORLD, infinitely complex and self-knowing, is starting to unfold in your womb, but you are not conscious of it yet. The Big Bang of your pregnancy will be undetectable for the next two weeks. While you speculate and hope, an egg, round and mysterious, is traveling from your ovary into your fallopian tube. There it awaits the kiss of the victorious hero, the one among 500 million sperm destined to penetrate the enclosed egg and make you both, mother and father, immortal. While in this world you embrace and meld with your beloved, in the hidden spaces of your womb fireworks erupt from your meeting, dividing again and again into mirror images of your original creation imprint. Today many couples or same-sex couples must depend upon a surrogate mother or in-vitro fertilization. If this is your situation, remember that though this is not happening in your womb, it is happening in your spirit womb, which kabbalists call the *diyok'na*. Visualize the first unfoldings of your child as if it is growing in your physical womb and send it the same attention and love. Your energetic connection is so important! In your womb or spirit womb, hundreds of cells are soon clustering around a fluid-filled cavity called

57

a blastocyst, reflecting in compact DNA patterning the chosen gender, form, coloring, and personality of your future child. Already beginning to unfurl and blossom into manifestation, like a perfectly folded origami flower tossed in water, your child will take nine months to reach her maturity.

You do not know it yet, but already in the third week (in actual fact it is the first week; even though you haven't yet conceived, doctors count pregnancy starting from the end of your last period) the blastocyst has emerged from the fallopian tube into your womb and is busy implanting firm roots into your uterine lining. (During the in-vitro process you will receive the fertilized egg five days after it reaches the blastocyst stage.) Soon it will be burrowing in for its long haul inside your body. Once firmly attached to the upper wall of your uterus, it will split in two, becoming your embryo and the placenta that supplies it with oxygen and nutrients. To pump the extra oxygen your baby now requires, your heart will beat faster and you will be tired: the first sign that you are pregnant. Week four, you miss your period. The blastocyst folds into three layers that will become the different systems of your baby's body. The endoderm will transform into intestines, liver, and lungs; the mesoderm into muscle, bones, and kidneys; the ectoderm becomes the brain, nervous system, skin, and eyes. Week five, your baby's heart starts beating. It's official—you're pregnant! Your seminal dream of becoming a mother is about to be realized.

It is customary to separate the time of gestation into three trimesters. The first trimester, weeks 1 to 13, which we will address in this chapter, is the time of implantation and adjustment to another life growing inside you. The second trimester, weeks 14 to 26, is the time of growth and greater development. The third trimester, weeks 27 to 40, marks the coming to maturity of your fetus.

ANNUNCIATION DREAMS

To find out with certainty whether you are pregnant, buy a little testing stick at your local pharmacist. At the doctor's office, the stick becomes a urine specimen the size of a big thimble. Both devices measure human chorionic gonadotrophin or hCG, a hormone only present when you are pregnant. The color appearing on the stick or in the cup, pink or blue, is the exciting confirmation you were waiting for. I remember the nurse coming out to the waiting room to show me the blue dot at the bottom of the cup. "You're pregnant, my dear!" I wasn't expecting it. I sobbed for five minutes with shock and the release of a tension I didn't even know I was carrying. I still have that little cup with the blue dot.

Why was I surprised? I had had, like many other mothers before me, my very own Annunciation dreams. Dreams tell us what the body is doing long before it can be measured on a little stick or in a cup. My first Annunciation dream telling me that I was pregnant—a night visitation, like the visitation of Archangel Gabriel to the Virgin Mary or that of the white elephant to Queen Maya, future mother of the Buddha—occurred at what turned out later to have been my time of conception.

I am in a thatched hut on a tiny island in the Caribbean Sea. The water surrounding the island is very blue. The four winds come blowing in, becoming one great being wearing the tall hat of his function, Gabriel the messenger. He becomes a twirling blue spiral at the center of the hut. I feel inhabited. I awake happy and fulfilled.

My second dream was a playful word dream. French is my native language. The word used in the dream was *l'enceinte d'une ville circonscrite,* the walls of a fortified city. *Enceinte* is also French for being pregnant.

A rabbi, wearing the fur hat and silk robes of the Hassidim, breaks through a postern gate in the wall of the fortified city— *l'enceinte de la ville circonscrite.*

The dream was telling me I was pregnant *(enceinte),* and circumcision *(circonscrite)* was to be expected. I would have a boy. The dream turned out to be a true prophecy. I dreamed those two dreams before I knew I had missed my period!

How is this possible? Dreams are messengers from the subconscious. Like undercurrent waves, they rise to the surface carrying messages from our subconscious long before our conscious mind is even aware that something is happening.

Pay attention to your dreams; they are your evening news bulletin. Free of charge, they inform you, showing you in images and words how your body, your emotions, and your baby are faring.

Have you had an Annunciation dream? Look back at your recent dreams and reflect. Wouldn't it be exciting to recognize that you had one? Or, if you are reading this in anticipation of becoming pregnant, ask your dreams to send you such a dream, then make sure to write down all your dreams, even those that appear to be the least significant or just snippets of dreams. You will be amazed at what your dreams tell you.

RESPOND TO THE NEEDS OF YOUR DREAMS

As your child grows in your womb, your dreams will become more intense, vivid, and specific. Why is that? Because you are secreting many more hormones when you are pregnant, and a steady influx of hormones enables you to remember your dreams. While hormone imbalance will affect your sleep and therefore your dreaming, women dream more vividly before ovulation and during pregnancy. At menopause, many women complain of diminished dream recall. Their dreams will return to them if they do something to boost their hormonal production. My Chinese doctor calls his hormone supplements "dream pills." You don't need dream pills because you are being flooded with hormones that help you and your child settle in together.

Write your dreams in your Dream Book. Your written records will allow you to verify whether your dreams turn out to have been true precursors of the future. Be sure to write any verifying facts in the margin next to your dream, using red ink. By systematically verifying the truthful outcome of your dreams in your everyday reality, you will have proved to yourself that you can trust your dreams. You will have proved that you can provide yourself, through your dreams, with a fast and precise diagnostic tool. This will allow you to anticipate both your body's and your baby's needs.

When your dreams are showing you that something is out of order or needs adjustment, respond to the need the images are indicating. Don't wait for symptoms to appear. For instance, if you were dreaming last night about standing on a patch of parched land, write your dream in your Dream Book and do the following exercise.

FACING THE NEEDS OF YOUR DREAM
exercise 26

Close your eyes. Breathe out slowly three times, counting from 3 to 1, seeing the numbers in your mind's eye. See the number 1 as tall, clear, and bright.

Returning to your dream, imagine that you use a garden hose to water the dry land, soaking it thoroughly. Do this until the land becomes moist and dark.

Breathe out. Open your eyes, seeing the moist land with open eyes.

Responding to the needs of your dreams is an effective way of talking to your body. By engaging with your dream images to restore harmony, you are actively stimulating your physical body to address the imbalance your dreams have diagnosed. In other words, you can use your dreams both as diagnosis and treatment. After responding through images to your dream needs, do not forget to also respond in your everyday reality. In this case, the message would be to make sure to drink more fluids!

Dream needs are like everyday needs. If you don't take responsibility, the situation gets worse. It is the same in the dream world: if the toilet is clogged, you use a plunger to unclog it. If your window is dirty, you wash it. If an intruder tries to break in, you call the police. But in the dream world, you are your own police. So weave a bulletproof jacket using sunbeams, put it on, open the door, and find out what the person wants. You may be surprised: All the intruder wants, usually, is some attention. Consider the intruder a messenger. If you dream that your baby's cord is wrapped around his neck, use your dream hands, filled with sunlight, to go in and free the cord (see *Loosen the cord,* exercise 98, page 179).

Your body talks to you in images. By responding in images, you ask your body to correct the imbalance. You will, of course, have to test what I am saying by doing the exercises yourself and checking the results. Nothing is more convincing than verifying for yourself. If you follow the program, you will have many occasions to confirm the effectiveness of using images to talk to your body.

PARADOXICAL FEELINGS

Your child has begun her journey to incarnation. You have been told so by your dreams. It has been confirmed by your pregnancy test and now by your doctor. Are you feeling excited and aware of the growing embryo in your womb? Or do you feel removed, disconnected from what is happening to you, maybe even a little frightened? Does this all feel too abstract for you?

This wouldn't be unusual in our fast-track modern world where the feeling person, even among females, is not extolled. Women in competitive jobs or stressful situations haven't the mind-set or leisure to examine their emotions. They are not encouraged or helped, especially in the US, to pursue both a career and motherhood. Stubbornly ignoring the inner messages from their unborn children and their own bodies, they will rush until the very last minute to finish whatever projects they are engaged in while resenting and fearing the fact that an infant, albeit theirs, will interrupt their momentum. These are the women who may later find it hard to adapt to their infant's needs.

Being focused on the outer world makes sense, it seems, if one wants to succeed in the world. But often what makes sense to our logical left brain is not necessarily what is most efficient. Succeeding in the workplace is not the only form of success worth pursuing.

The news that you are going to have a baby cannot fail to strike a deep chord, even in the most disconnected. You have stepped onto a new shore, but nothing is visible as yet. No wonder you feel suspended, uprooted, unsure. Your life will never be the same again. Even if you planned this pregnancy, you cannot help but mourn for what is lost, while feeling apprehension about the new form life will take. The shock of suddenly knowing you are inhabited by another life is prodding you toward introspection. Let this thrill of sensations happen.

Take the time to feel. Your conflicting emotions, if you allow them to coexist within, can only enrich you. Enjoy your garden of paradox.

THE GARDEN OF PARADOX
exercise 27

Close your eyes. Breathe out slowly three times, counting from 3 to 1, seeing the numbers in your mind's eye. See the number 1 as tall, clear, and bright.

Looking into a full-length mirror, sense, see, and feel that you are now carrying a child.

Breathe out. In the mirror, see a flower appearing for each one of your different emotions. Name your emotions.

Breathe out. Once you have all your flowers, look at the bouquet you are holding and discard the flowers that don't fit, sweeping them out of the mirror to your left, using your left hand.

Breathe out. When you are satisfied with the way your bouquet looks, put your hand in the mirror and pull out the bouquet, bringing it to your nose to smell its fragrance. What are you feeling? What has changed?

Breathe out. Open your eyes, seeing the bouquet with open eyes.

We will be dealing at greater length with the different emotions and conflicting thoughts that may appear during your pregnancy. For the moment it is good simply to be able to feel what you feel—and not judge yourself for your feelings. Staying alone with your emotions may not be a good idea. Find someone trustworthy you can talk to, such as your partner, your mother, your therapist, or a supportive older woman or friend who's already gone through pregnancy: people who can provide useful insights into what you are experiencing and reassure you that your intensified state of feeling is quite common in pregnancy. Ignoring your inner processes would only lead you to ignore the growing life within your womb.

GREETING YOUR CHILD

Now that you are feeling more aware and, hopefully, more accepting of your feelings, it's time to turn your attention to the new life that is just beginning to unfold in your womb.

Think of it. Your baby is growing inside of you. You are her first environment, the ocean in which she swims. Every change in you registers as a ripple or a storm in that ocean. Every experience you have affects her. Your baby is not developed enough to be verbally conscious, but she *is* experientially conscious. Your baby senses and feels. She is physiologically in tune with you. While your impact is on her body, not her conscious mind, remember that her right brain registers as dream patterns whatever is happening in her body. If these dream patterns are acute or repetitive, later on in life she will be able to access them and translate them into conscious thought.

Many studies have shown that your baby is learning in the womb. Researchers are still uncertain when memory begins, but it is certain that five weeks into your pregnancy (in fact two weeks of actual gestation), your baby is already reacting to outside stimuli. Faint or detailed traces of memory have been recorded through hypnosis of the adult-child and verified by appealing directly to the mother for corroboration. Through guided imagery I have often taken people back into the womb and asked them to describe what they were feeling at four months gestation, at three, at the moment of conception. For the most part, they have no trouble doing so. Whenever possible, we have obtained verification. Many studies since the early 1970s have shown incontestable evidence that your unborn child, from very early on in her gestation, is a sentient, feeling being.

We don't exist in a vacuum and your child doesn't either. She is in a relationship with you and, through you, with the environment you live in, the larger world, and even the cosmos. So your attitude toward your unborn child is the single most important factor in determining how your baby will develop in your uterus and after she is born. If you are accepting and loving of her, if you pay attention to her as she develops, and if you reassure her when something has upset her in the process of upsetting you, your child will thrive. She will be healthier both physically and emotionally. Since, as studies have shown, she can sense her mother's attention or rejection of her from the very first weeks, the earlier and more finely attuned you are to the new life in your womb, the better it will be for your baby and you.

So how do you communicate with this invisible entity inside you? You may naturally start talking to your little one. Or you may find this strange or uncomfortable, more so if you know that babies' hearing only develops by the 16th week of gestation. However, any form of loving interaction between you and your baby is important. Talking, singing, sending sweet images, and caressing your womb are manifestations of loving attention. Turning your eyes inward to *see* inside your body is the strongest way of communicating. Your body language is images. The language your baby understands best at this early stage of development is images. What you experience through images affects you in a more visceral way than simply thinking about an outcome.

The following exercise is your most important pregnancy exercise. You should practice it every day of your pregnancy until your 32nd week, when you will begin to practice a different exercise called *Rehearsing the birth*.

Do this one to three times a day. I recommend that you practice this exercise at midday, then rest for a half hour before continuing your day. Resting is essential to your and your child's well-being.

For this exercise, you will need to refer to a chart that shows you how the fetus develops week by week. You will find many versions of the chart on the Internet. Each week, check to see what is developing in your baby and visualize it growing perfectly. For example, if the villi (the roots of the placenta) are implanting into the wall of your uterus, see them implanting deeply; if your baby is developing fingers, visualize those fingers growing perfectly.

The exercise is good for second- and multiple-time moms and moms who are expecting twins. Instead of one baby, just visualize two. You can talk to the two or to one baby at a time. The exercise soothes, calms, and harmonizes your body for the perfect unfolding of your unborn child. It also prepares both you and your child for an easy birth.

If you have had a shock or are upset, your body rhythms will change and will affect your unborn child. Do this exercise as soon as possible afterward. Your baby needs to be reassured.

GOING INTO THE WOMB
TO VISIT YOUR CHILD
exercise 28

Close your eyes. Breathe out slowly three times, counting from 3 to 1, seeing the numbers in your mind's eye. See the number 1 as tall, clear, and bright.

Turn your eyes inward to travel down to your womb. Your eyes shine like two beams illuminating your way down inside your body to the amniotic sac. When you are there, bring your eyes close to the transparent membrane of the sac and look at your baby floating freely in its clear blue amniotic waters.

Breathe out. Talk to your baby (later on, when your baby has reached the stage of development when her eyes are open, make eye contact with her while talking). Tell your baby all you want to tell her, using words or images. Tell her how much you love her, how much you are looking forward to her arrival.

Breathe out. Tell her of any particular stresses or shocks you may be experiencing. Tell her not to worry, that all is well, that she's safe inside the amniotic sac, tucked under your heart.

Breathe out. Remind your baby of the particular phase of development she's in right now (according to the chart) and visualize the perfect development of that part of her body. (Remember that the phase changes each week, so keep in touch with the weekly changes and visualize them happening perfectly.)

Breathe out. Tell your baby you have to go now but that you'll be back to visit again at lunch and dinner times. Tell her that even though you may be busy with other things, she's safely in your body and being taken care of.

Breathe out. Bring your eyes back up into your sockets.

Breathe out. Open your eyes, registering the room around you while also seeing with open eyes your baby tucked comfortably under your heart.

Keep visualizing your child's unfolding manifestation until your child is able to take full responsibility for her life. "Only by way of the Image shall a person journey."[15] This process of imagination does not end with birth, but continues throughout your child's life. Until your child reaches maturity, you are responsible for holding in your mind's eye only the most positive, life-affirming images for her. This does not mean that you see your child through rose-tinted lenses but that, while being perfectly cognizant of what reality holds for your child, you project for her only the very best. Eventually the responsibility for creating her own healthy unfolding becomes her own.

The old teachings tell us that creation is happening right now, that every blade of grass is being brought forth into being at every moment by the Creator's imagination.[16] So, too, like the blade of grass, to be fully and powerfully brought into being, your creation requires your devotional love and focus. This will be your work as cocreators.

Note that even the father's attitudes toward the pregnancy affect the development of your child in the womb and after birth. The father, with some variations, can also do this exercise (see chapter 8, page 253).

EXHAUSTED? NEEDING A PICK-ME-UP?

There is an ancient kabbalistic theory that at the moment of the Big Bang, the Divine removes Himself to make room for His creation. He becomes the mother to His creation. He creates a womblike space into which the forms He has dreamed may unfold. In the same way, you, the mother, are the Divine to your child creation. Like a matryoshka, a Russian nesting doll, you nest in the Divine and your child nests in you.

Did the Divine Mother have growing pains as today's mothers do? Was She fatigued or nauseous? Did She become irritable and weepy, maybe even irrational? Making space is difficult, and accommodating another mouth to feed is stressful. So do not believe, as did one of my young students, that if you are suddenly extremely exhausted or nauseous, you must be ill. She was afraid to talk about it because she was sure that something was very wrong with her baby and that she was to blame. Being fatigued is normal; being nauseous happens to more than half the pregnant population. You are *not* ill.

While you are blind to what is really going on inside of you (until you learn to dream!), your body is sentient. It knows itself, communicates cell to cell, organ to organ, and it participates in setting up the new program put in motion by the fertilization of your egg. The blastocyst—the hollow ball of cells formed from the division of the original cell into two, four, eight, sixteen cells, becoming the morula when cells begin to differentiate—has descended into the uterus. There, the blastocyst's inner cells begin forming the embryo and amniotic sac while its outer cells burrow into the lining of your uterus, becoming the placenta. It is the placenta that is your baby's life-support system.

From the very beginning, your baby's placenta produces the hormone called human chorionic gonadotrophin, which prevents ovaries from producing eggs while stimulating them to continually pump out estrogen and progesterone. So much hormonal activity and cell growth within your womb are bound to make you feel tired, irritable, maybe even a little weepy.

Your body is far more intelligent than your mind is. By bringing on the deep exhaustion that is typical of early pregnancy, your body is saying, "Please rest!" Don't spend your precious quota of energy on extraneous activities. Think of what happens when you have eaten a big meal. You feel sleepy because all your resources of energy are co-opted to help your digestive system cope with the extra load of food. During pregnancy, your body is being asked to set up a whole new infrastructure and to maintain it at the same time. No wonder you're tired!

There is a simple way to boost your energy. Remember that you are not alone in the world. You are in constant interaction with nature. This next exercise may remind you of the *Conception exercise* (page 50) in which you sit under a big tree. It is based on photosynthesis, the process by which vegetation, using the energy of the sun, converts the carbon dioxide we exhale into organic compounds and exudes oxygen, which we breathe in. We depend on vegetation for the oxygen in our atmosphere.

BREATHING WITH THE TREE
exercise 29

Close your eyes. Breathe out slowly three times, counting from 3 to 1, seeing the numbers in your mind's eye. See the 1 as tall, clear, and bright.

Imagine that you are looking up at an emerald-green hill upon which stands a magnificent tree. Describe the tree to yourself.

Breathe out. Walk up to the tree. Sit under the tree, your baby safely tucked under your heart, your back against the tree trunk, your knees bent. Sink your toes into the rich soil and feel them becoming long roots. Sink your fingers into the soil and feel them becoming long roots.

Slowly breathe out a light smoke, like a cigarette smoke, containing all that tires you, all that obscures you, all that upsets you. See the light smoke rising up into the canopy of the tree and being absorbed by its leaves.

See yourself breathing in the oxygen the tree releases.

See this great ring of breathing that links you and your baby with the tree.

As you continue breathing, see the sap rising up the roots through the trunk of the tree and your spine. See its color.

Continue breathing until you feel replenished.

Breathe out. Lift up your toes and fingers, get up, and step away from your tree. Turn around and look at the tree. What, if anything, has changed in the tree and in you?

Breathe out. If your tree looks in any way depleted, go to the small river that runs nearby and, filling a container of water, water your tree. Step back and see what happens. If you are still not satisfied with the way your tree looks, water it again until you are satisfied that both you and your tree have been enriched by the encounter.

Breathe out. Walk down the grassy hill, feeling invigorated.

Breathe out. Open your eyes.

You can practice this exercise in your home—even better, sitting near a green plant or outside under a tree. You can practice it as many times a day as you like but not longer than three minutes at a time. Don't practice it at night before going to bed. Since it increases your oxygen consumption, it might keep you awake.

MORNING SICKNESS, A PHENOMENON OF ADJUSTMENT

There is nothing romantic about morning sickness, the nausea and occasional vomiting that can occur during pregnancy. The term is a misnomer, as it may affect you morning, noon, or night and is not really a sickness. We could call it a phenomenon of adjustment. In most cases, it disappears promptly at the end of the third month. Some women continue to suffer episodically in the second and third trimesters. A rare few experience it throughout their pregnancy. There are different degrees of nausea, from mild queasiness to intense vomiting. More than 50 percent of pregnant women get morning sickness, so if you are among the lucky ones not affected, consider yourself blessed.

Why do pregnant women get morning sickness? No one knows for sure, although there are many theories involving higher levels of estrogen and progesterone as well as maternal serum prostaglandin E2 levels in the blood, relaxation of the muscle tissues of the digestive tract, and enhanced sense of smell. Morning sickness may have an evolutionary reason as well: keeping pregnant women from eating meats and pungent vegetables that could harm the fetus. In traditional cultures where animal foods are not consumed, morning sickness is practically nonexistent. Morning sickness seems to affect more women during their first pregnancy when they are unprepared for the onslaught of hormones and are prone to the anxieties and fears of the novice mother. Women who are under stress, or who are not happy about being pregnant, also are more prone to it, suggesting that there are emotional as well as physical causes involved.

This makes sense. When you are frightened, anxious, or stressed, you get an upset stomach. Since the brain stem is the neurological center for control of nausea and vomiting, your first exercise for nausea will be to learn how to calm your brain stem nausea control center. Remember that images are the language of the body. You can use them to interact with the involuntary functions of your body.

INDIGO COLUMN
exercise 30

Close your eyes. Breathe out slowly three times, counting from 3 to 1, seeing the numbers in your mind's eye. See the number 1 as tall, clear, and bright.

Imagine that it is nighttime and you are sitting outside, enveloped in the restful, warm, indigo-blue night.

Breathe out. Feel the night all around you, and sense the back of your neck resting against the night sky. See your neck becoming indigo blue like the night, and wider and longer, like a wide, tall indigo-blue column. What do you sense and feel in your body?

Breathe out. Open your eyes, feeling this with open eyes.

You can also directly train your stomach not to react by using colors that are soothing and calming for the digestive system. As color and its associated memories are particular to each individual, choose your own colors.

CLEARING COLOR
exercise 31

Close your eyes. Breathe out slowly three times, counting from 3 to 1, seeing the numbers in your mind's eye. See the number 1 as tall, clear, and bright.

Turning your eyes inward to your stomach, see the color of your upset stomach.

Breathe out. Sweep this color out of your body to the left, using your left hand.

Breathe out. Permeate your stomach with the color that is the very opposite color from the one you have swept away. If you can't find the opposite color, choose turquoise. What do you feel now? If the color is soothing to your stomach, ask your body to keep it there for the next twenty-four hours.

Breathe out. Open your eyes, seeing the color with open eyes.

NORMAL CAUSES OF ANXIETY—CLEARING THE WAY

Pregnancy brings with it both the relief of knowing you have made it to pregnancy and many new anxieties. If you are a first-time mom, you don't really know what to expect. You may be worrying about your fatigue, your nausea, your enlarged breasts, your increased need to urinate, the spotting that can sometimes occur early on in a pregnancy, the changes your body is going through. You may be wrestling with many questions: How will I handle labor? What kind of mother will I be? Will I be able to recover my figure after the birth? Will my partner adapt to our changed circumstances? Will he/she still love me? How will a child impact our relationship, our way of life, our finances? How or when will I announce the news at work?

As you know, stress is not good for your body, and it's not good for your baby. But how does one handle stress? There are a few trusted ways, such as informing yourself through books and tapes and talking to your mother, another reliable older female, or friends who have gone through a successful pregnancy. Knowing what to expect makes it easier.

Do not listen to those who will want to regale you with horror stories. They will only make you more anxious and impact your body in a negative way. The old wives' tale of surrounding pregnant women with calm, serenity, and beauty has been proven true by modern studies. And you now have your own tool, dream exercises, to dialogue with your body in a serene way and elicit from it the very best outcome. Here's another exercise to try.

THE COCOON OF LIGHT
exercise 32

Close your eyes. Breathe out slowly three times, counting from 3 to 1, seeing the numbers in your mind's eye. See the number 1 as tall, clear, and bright.

Imagine that you stretch your arm up toward the sun and catch a ray of light.

Breathe out. Draw a cocoon of light from your feet right up to your head, enveloping yourself and your baby. Know that no unwelcome person or voice can penetrate that cocoon of protection.

Breathe out. Open your eyes, seeing the cocoon of light around you and your baby.

When no longer in need of protection, remove the cocoon of light and return the ray to the sun. You can do this with open eyes.

Remember that your thoughts, emotions, and images directly affect your body. This is why, for the sake of your baby, you must exercise your mind, emotions, and images toward the greater calm, serenity, and beauty that old wives recommended for pregnant women. Each time you sweep away an obsessive thought, a difficult emotion (fear, anger, resentment, guilt), or a negative image and replace it with a healthy thought, feeling, or image, you are creating for yourself the positive environment that will benefit you and your baby.

SWEEP THE PORCH
exercise 33

Close your eyes. Breathe out slowly three times, counting from 3 to 1, seeing the numbers in your mind's eye. See the number 1 as tall, clear, and bright.

See yourself standing on the porch of an old country house. The porch is covered with dry leaves.

Breathe out. Take a garden broom and sweep the dry leaves off the porch to the left. Experience all the physical sensations of sweeping.

Breathe out. See that the porch is now clean; there isn't a single leaf left. What are you feeling?

Breathe out. Open your eyes.

It is worth noting the strange Bible story of the solid-colored flocks of sheep and goats that, by staring at striped branches while they mated, bore striped young.[17] Can what we look at actually affect our baby's DNA? At this point, no one knows. But we do know that what we see affects our bodies. We blush, our heart beats speed up, we are sexually aroused, we tremble with fear—all from reacting to what we see. So it is important to know how to deal with what you see, especially when it provokes fear.

WASHING AWAY FEARS
exercise 34

Close your eyes. Breathe out slowly three times, counting from 3 to 1, seeing the numbers in your mind's eye. See the number 1 as tall, clear, and bright.

In a mirror, see the image of your fear.

Breathe out. Wash that image out of the mirror to the left with your left hand.

Breathe out. Look into the mirror and see what gives you joy.

Breathe out. Open your eyes, keeping the image of your joy preciously in your heart.

"SEEING" YOUR BABY FOR THE FIRST TIME

Your second visit to your obstetrician will be at 7 weeks' gestation. If you are working with a doctor, as opposed to a midwife, he or she will perform a routine sonogram that will allow you to "see" your baby for the first time on a monitor (you have already seen her with your inner eyes). She is tiny and doesn't yet look human. But you will hear your baby's heartbeat for the first time!

Between 18 and 20 weeks, a second sonogram is routinely administered, during which you will have the thrill of seeing your baby floating in the amniotic sac. It now looks like a real baby—with hands and fingers; feet and toes; eyes, nose, and mouth; the beginning of ears; some hair on the head; and female genitalia or a penis! You will even be able to see baby moving!

What are sonograms, otherwise called ultrasound imaging? They are images produced by very high frequency sound waves (3.5 to 7.0 megahertz) emitted from a transducer through the skin of the abdomen covered in gel. The gel works as a conductor for the sound waves. As the transducer is moved across your abdomen, the sound waves bounce off your baby's body and generate images on a monitor screen. This allows the doctor to measure fetal growth and scan for any complications. Meanwhile, you and your partner are peeking into the Garden of Eden, something no one had ever done before the 1960s. When you leave the doctor's office, you're presented with a picture of your baby that you can later show to your family members and friends. It is all very exciting. Many doctors now routinely use the sonogram when you come in for your prenatal visits.

At the risk of being unpopular, I am compelled to question whether ultrasound imaging is safe. While your doctor may tell you there is no danger, the FDA warned in 2004 that "ultrasound is a form of energy, and even at low levels, laboratory studies have shown it can produce physical effects in tissue, such as jarring vibrations and a rise in temperature." A rise in fetal tissue temperature has been shown to affect neuronal migration in mice, and the damage was consistent with that found in the brain tissues of people with autism.[18] While your baby will not be receiving as lengthy an application of ultrasounds as the mice (thirty-five minutes), she is a developing fetus being subjected to ultra-high-frequency sound waves just as her brain and body are being formed. Is this even necessary? The National Institutes of Health recommends that ultrasound imaging during pregnancy not be used for routine screening but only where specific medical need is indicated. This is also the position of the American College of Obstetricians and Gynecologists.

Even if you don't agree that there are strong reasons to question repeated use of sonograms during a routine pregnancy (I hope you will do your own research on ultrasound imaging; fetal monitoring also uses ultrasound, so don't forget to do your research there too), please do this simple protection exercise if and when you do have a sonogram. It takes at most thirty seconds.

WHITE SCREEN
exercise 35

Close your eyes. Breathe out slowly three times, counting from 3 to 1, seeing the numbers in your mind's eye. See the number 1 as tall, clear, and bright.

Looking up at the radiant sky, stretch your arms up to catch a screen of the most radiant white light and pull it down over your body and baby.

Breathe out. Feel how the screen protects you from all outside interference and ask that it continue to protect you as long as is needed. What do you experience when your body is protected by the screen of light?

Breathe out. Open your eyes, seeing the screen of light with open eyes. Let go of the screen when you no longer need to be protected.

Technology has many pluses, but no one can doubt that it also has its drawbacks. Unfortunately, it often takes time for the damaging effects of technology to accumulate so that they become clear enough for everyone to acknowledge them. So I will take another unpopular position and advocate against having cell phones next to your body. This also includes cordless phones. A collaborative study done at UCLA and in Aarhus, Denmark, involving thirteen thousand children, showed that mothers using handsets were 54 percent more likely to have children with behavioral problems. When those children used cell phones later, they were 80 percent more likely to have behavioral problems. The European Union, recognizing the risk to children, has banned all cell phones and cell towers near schools (we are slower in the United States to consider giving up or curtailing our use of cell phones). Is it the radiation that adversely affects children and adults? The answers aren't in yet, but, according to a Canadian study, structural changes have been found in the offspring of pregnant rats exposed to similar radiation. Considering the rising percentage of children with behavioral or constitutional problems, wouldn't it be wiser to play it safe? In fact, wouldn't it be a good idea—to protect our fertility, personal health, and longevity—to make it a lifelong habit to keep our cell phones away from our bodies?

If you read these cautionary remarks "too late" in the unfolding process of your pregnancy, remember what I said at the end of the introduction. The subconscious is ever present and ever malleable. Practice *Going into the womb to visit your child* (page 66), seeing your child developing perfectly. If needed, your "seeing" will repair whatever has to be repaired. Trust in the power of your "seeing."

ENDING THE FIRST TRIMESTER

You are coming to the end of the first trimester. The nausea and fatigue are diminishing. (If your nausea persists, which happens in a small percentage of women, continue doing the exercises for nausea, cut fatty foods from your diet, and follow your doctor's or midwife's advice). Overnight, it seems, you are feeling much more energetic and want to be more active. At the same time, you're getting bigger, and you feel the need for safety and protection. You and your baby have gotten through this first lap of your journey. You want to cherish your newfound well-being and optimism within the cocoon of your pregnancy. This exercise will help transition you to the next segment of your journey.

THE CHALICE
exercise 36

Close your eyes. Breathe out slowly three times, counting from 3 to 1, seeing the numbers in your mind's eye. See the number 1 as tall, clear, and bright.

Imagine that you are sitting under a tree on thick emerald-green grass.

Breathe out. See appearing in front of you a large golden chalice filled to the brim with precious stones of every color.

Breathe out. Watch as the sunlight touches the stones, brightening all the colors.

Breathe out. See the colors spreading to envelop you and your baby, creating a many-colored aura around both of you. Feel it soothing, healing, protecting you.

Breathe out. Open your eyes, seeing the aura with your eyes open.

Beauty and soothing colors are what every pregnant woman needs. Allow your partner to pamper you. Don't be afraid to ask for what you need, whether it's help with cleaning, shopping, or cooking or that you need a beautiful new dress. Remember that your partner wants to participate. Allowing him (or her) to spoil you to his (or her) heart's content is doing him (or her) a favor. Pregnant women's cravings are legendary so don't be afraid to indulge. And of course, don't forget to ask for more TLC if you need it. After all, you're carrying the family treasure, and you're entitled.

4

Basking in the Glow

Life is always a rich and steady time when you are
waiting for something to happen or to hatch.

E. B. WHITE

YOU HAVE REACHED the long-awaited milestone of your fourth month. For many, this feels like emerging out of a dark, dank place into the sunshine. Just when you were feeling that you couldn't bear your misery any longer, it ceases! One day you wake up raring to go. The queasiness is mostly gone. What has happened? Remember the pregnancy hormone hCG that, linked to increased levels of estrogen, is believed to cause nausea? When the fetus is firmly established within the uterus, this hormone decreases and so does your queasiness. Suddenly you are feeling active and healthy again, feeling like yourself for the first time since learning that your baby was growing inside you. Your baby's placenta, his home within the sky of your body, is now firmly rooted in the lining of your uterus. This is your golden age when sun and moon are co-partnering to make you look radiantly healthy and mysteriously luminous, just like the Mona Lisa. (Was she pregnant? She looks secretive, like the cat that swallowed the canary. And so will you this trimester as you shine and glow with contentment.)

81

Already you can no longer hide the waxing of your moonlike belly. It will continue to grow until, like Selene, the Greek goddess of the moon, you will see yourself as the full moon reflected in the dark waters of the night. Like her, you are becoming larger than life, wiser, deeper, untouchable, and, like the Creation Mother herself, both familiar and strange. Enjoy this time, as your radiance and the fruit it bears will give both of you immunity from all physical exertions and the prerogative of having any of your cravings, however irrational, immediately met. You are not required to do anything but let the seed grow in you. Don't try to be a superwoman; just let yourself be cared for.

The baby growing in you is reflective of the sun's benevolence, how the sun is such a nourishing and life-enhancing force for all of life. The sun's radiance and bounty are then reflected back by the moon to all living organisms. We see this manifested in a surge of hormones, hyperpigmenting the areolas around your nipples and, in some cases, spotting or masking your face with discolorations (they fade after delivery). The white line descending from your navel to your pubic bone turns black. It is called the *linea negra*. As these and other signs appear on your body, you are morphing into the mysterious Black Madonna, hugging her secret fruit in her dark recesses, like Eve, whose name signifies mother of all living.

ADAPTING TO THE CHANGES IN YOUR BODY

Your first three months will probably turn out to be the most taxing of your pregnancy, which is good news as you enter your second trimester. By this time, your body is beginning to show signs of pregnancy. You may marvel at what your body is able to accomplish. You will enjoy showing off the roundness of your belly to friends who want to rejoice with you. Or you may worry about your body image and changing form: Will I be able to return to my former trim self? Will those faint new stretch marks worsen? Will they disappear after the birth? Will my partner be turned off? Am I becoming repugnant to myself? Meanwhile, your doctor's warning about not putting on too much weight may be raising red flags for you. These anxieties about your body image can be very painful, especially if you live in a culture that reveres slimness. If you live in more rural or tribal societies that cherish the roundness of pregnancy, you will be spared these worries.

Your happiness about yourself and with yourself is important for your well-being and that of your growing fetus. Though your body image is in flux at all times, this is one of those periods when the changes are more pronounced. Recognize that these are not permanent changes. You will grow larger throughout your pregnancy; then, after the birth, you will get trimmer again. So take time to enjoy the roundness and newfound softness that amplify your femininity. In chapter 7 you will find more exercises to help you to find the natural body size and image that make you feel good about yourself.

BODY CYCLES
exercise 37

Close your eyes. Breathe out slowly three times, counting from 3 to 1, seeing the numbers in your mind's eye. See the number 1 as tall, clear, and bright.

Imagine that you are walking deep into the woods on a bright, sunny day. Feel the dappled sunlight and the breeze on your skin; listen to the sounds of nature.

Breathe out. Come to an opening where a full-length mirror is awaiting you. See yourself in the mirror as you are just now.

Breathe out. See your shape changing as you grow through your pregnancy. If you feel that the change shows too much weight gain, sweep the image off to the left and see yourself in the mirror having gained exactly what is appropriate for that moment in your pregnancy.

Breathe out. Continue seeing and adjusting the changes until the moment of birth.

Breathe out. See your baby in your arms. Place your baby in a bower of green grass.

Breathe out. Continue looking into the mirror. See your body going through the stages of losing its roundness until it becomes firm and energetic. Continue looking until you are perfectly satisfied.

Breathe out. See in the mirror the date at which you will be perfectly satisfied.

Breathe out. Caress your rounded belly with your two hands, sending love to your child and knowing that throughout your pregnancy, you will gain at any given time the appropriate amount of weight, and that when your baby is born, you will be able to return to a perfectly firm and energetic form.

Breathe out. Open your eyes, seeing the transformation with open eyes.

Remember that your subconscious is programmed by your images and that those images command your body. If you feel negative about yourself, your body will conform. So graciously and joyfully accept the changes of your pregnant body while consciously imagining the look you want to have after your baby is born. You can do this exercise whenever you feel uneasy about the way you look as a pregnant woman. You are already setting the intent to return to your natural form. Intent is very powerful; your body will respond when the time comes.

Take pleasure in your changing form. You might even choose to get yourself some comfortable and chic maternity clothes so you can feel fashionable and elegant.

REALITY AND WORRIES ABOUT EXPECTING

Now that you are showing, there can be no doubt in your mind or anyone else's that you are pregnant. With the inexorable growth of the baby in your womb, you are faced with the reality that, in six months' time, you will give birth. You will become a parent.

You may be shouting for joy, and even as you are singing your hallelujahs, having moments of apprehension. You may feel trapped, which is quite natural. These are the first signs of your developing a feeling of responsibility, not for yourself but for the defenseless being you are carrying. If you haven't yet learned to forget yourself for another, that is where nature challenges you. Caring for a child teaches selflessness and compassion. You will have to put your child's needs before your own. But don't worry: you'll learn to love in this selfless way as you go along.

Your baby is rapidly growing and morphing within the purview of the moon. He will grow fuzz all over his body, just as grass grows on the surface of the earth. He will consolidate his bones into a treelike structure. He will begin the inner stretching out to touch, hear, taste, smell, see. Throughout his life, his senses will continue their adventurous tracking. We call this movement "longing."

As your baby develops his blueprint according to a clocked timetable, you naturally want to know whether all is unfolding according to plan. Now that your energy is freed from the all-consuming effort of adjusting to a foreign body, you have more leisure to listen to your inner voices. You may return to destructive old habits or find yourself assailed by familiar voices of worry and doubt. We are never completely immune to catastrophic voices—until we learn to be in the Now.

CLEARING CATASTROPHIC VOICES
exercise 38

Close your eyes. Breathe out slowly three times, counting from
3 to 1, seeing the numbers in your mind's eye. See the number
1 as tall, clear, and bright.

Listen to your catastrophic voice. From what direction does it come? From your left, left back, right, right back—where?

Breathe out. Stretch your arm up toward the sun, catch a ray of light, and surround yourself with light. Once protected, turn to face the voice and see who is talking.

Breathe out. Lift up a large conelike structure in the direction of the voice. Capture the sounds in the cone and see them resonating back to the person who produced them.

Breathe out. Push the cone away from you into space toward the person, until the cone, the sounds, and the person disappear completely.

Breathe out. Listen to the silence. Enjoy it.

Breathe out. Open your eyes.

Once you have cleared out of your field the one whose voice was invading you, you still have to learn to deal with the bad habit. Your body is a creature of habit, and it is used to hearing the voice. So don't be surprised if your body imitates the voice. But notice that it is not quite as intense and all-invasive. Bad habits—such as smoking, binge eating, drinking, anxiety, doubting or hating voices, to name only a few—are numerous and need to be swept away just as we would sweep away the dirt in our house.

SWEEPING AWAY BAD HABITS
exercise 39

Close your eyes. Breathe out slowly three times, counting from 3 to 1, seeing the numbers in your mind's eye. See the number 1 as tall, clear, and bright.

Take a small broom and sweep the voice off to the left.

Breathe out. Open your eyes.

You may have to continue sweeping for quite a long time. Habits are made over time and must be eradicated over time. So just sweep whenever the voice surfaces. If you do this faithfully, I can assure you that one day, the voice will be gone for good.

If the voice you are hearing is not someone else's but your own, remember that even your own unhealthy voices can "drive the bus." You can clear your unhealthy voices by doing the following exercise.

THE DARK CLOUD
exercise 40

Breathe out, seeing your exhalation as a dark smoke that gathers ahead and above you in the sky, becoming a dark cloud. Continue to breathe out the dark smoke, seeing the cloud get larger as you breathe out. Continue until your breath becomes clearer, then transparent.

Now breathe out strongly against the cloud, breaking it into thousands of pieces.

Breathe out a second time, seeing the pieces dissolving.

Breathe out a third time, seeing that all the wisps of smoke have disappeared, and the sky is very blue and clear.

Open your eyes, seeing the sky as very blue and clear.

This exercise works wonders for anxiety. Anxiety can be useful in prompting you to uncover the real cause of your stress. But if your anxiety has no real cause and feels overwhelming, it is time to do something about it. Practice this exercise regularly every morning for twenty-one days to teach your body to clean out the negative habit. If twenty-one days are not enough, stop for seven days and do another round of twenty-one days. In this way, you train yourself to break the habit of crippling anxiety. Perseverance makes a world of difference.

HOW TO COPE WITH TESTING

Even if you are not crippled with anxiety, you wouldn't be human if you didn't ask yourself the obvious questions: Is my baby healthy? Is he developing correctly? Should I be tested? Between the 16th and 18th weeks your doctor will be suggesting different tests to you, as he will want to check your baby's chromosomes, skin, and blood.

Before you decide to go ahead with testing, use the tools you have already learned. Remember that *Going into the womb to visit your child* (page 66) is your most important exercise. You are turning your eyes into your body to "see" your child. Trust your inner eyes: they are the tools of your *in*-tuition.

If your worries and doubts continue to cloud your inner vision, you can access your night dreams. It is easier to see the truth when your conscious mind is asleep. Before going to sleep remember to *Sweep the porch* (page 75) or your worries could invade your dreams and give you nightmares. Sometimes the nightmare is really trying to tell you something. In that case, remember that dreams are not only a diagnostic tool but also a therapeutic means of repairing what has gone awry. Take your dream seriously. Respond to its needs imaginally and, if necessary, call your doctor.

In most cases, your nightmare is only highlighting your anxiety. Your dream life gets much more intense when you're flooded with hormones. Your nightlife persona can suddenly metamorphose from reasonable woman to drama queen. Don't take her too seriously. Learn to recognize the difference between your drama queen dreams and precognitive dreams.

Not sure? Go back into the dream and ask: is this an anxious dream? You will hear the answer right away. Trust it. Long before your conscious mind becomes aware of any change in your body, your body, being the locus of happening, "knows." And it speaks to you through dreams and visions.

Still not convinced that you're just having an anxious dream? If you feel that testing will make you feel safer—or if your family background, medical history, or age warrant testing—by all means have the tests. But no test comes without risk. So you will need to prepare your baby and your body for the procedure.

The most common test at this stage is amniocentesis, which checks the fetal cells, chemicals, and microorganisms in the amniotic fluid. The doctor inserts a long, hollow needle through the abdominal wall into the uterus and withdraws amniotic fluid from your baby's sac. You will feel no pain when the needle is inserted. The doctor looks at the monitor screen to see where your baby is and inserts the needle as far away from the baby as possible (remember to do the *White screen* exercise, page 78, as a sonogram is involved). Don't forget to visualize your baby moving to one side of the amniotic sac until the procedure is over. He will respond to your internal image making. You will be able to verify this on the monitor screen.

❧

TO PREPARE FOR PROCEDURES
exercise 41

Close your eyes. Breathe out slowly three times, counting from 3 to 1, seeing the numbers in your mind's eye. See the number 1 as tall, clear, and bright.

Show your body in a precise visualization exactly what is going to happen and ask your body's permission to allow the procedure your doctor is about to perform.

Breathe out. If your body refuses permission, ask your body what it needs in order to accept the procedure. Respond to your body's needs in images.

Breathe out. Once your body has given permission, ask your baby's permission to allow the procedure.

Breathe out. If your baby refuses permission, ask your baby what he needs in order to accept the procedure. Respond to your baby's needs in images.

Breathe out. Do this until your body, your baby, and you are all in agreement about having the procedure.

❧

You will find a more complete version of the exercise, *The garden—to prepare for procedures,* in appendix 1, page 285. It combines this exercise with the *Secret garden* exercise (page 95).

It is normal to have a little cramping after amniocentesis. Here's what you do.

COLOR FOR CRAMPING
exercise 42

Close your eyes. Breathe out slowly three times, counting from 3 to 1, seeing the numbers in your mind's eye. See the number 1 as tall, clear, and bright.

For one minute visualize the color magenta in your lower back and lower abdomen.

Breathe out. Open your eyes, seeing the color with open eyes for a few seconds.[19]

Waiting for results can be emotional. You are all wound up, but in expectation of what? You know that you have faithfully practiced all your exercises. You know that your mind's vitalizing images positively affect your body and that of your child. Don't let your mind run away with "what ifs" and catastrophic or negative thoughts. Trust that the light guiding your feet on the path of well-being and happiness will not fail you and will guide you all the way. And don't forget to go back into the womb to visit with your child. That will reassure both of you that all is well.

The more you concentrate on your child's beauty and perfection, the more you help nature to perfect your creation. This is not a vain hope, but you will have to verify what I say through the following exercise. You are a co-creator with the Divine and with nature.

LADIES' HAPPINESS
exercise 43

Close your eyes. Breathe out slowly three times, counting from 3 to 1, seeing the numbers in your mind's eye. See the number 1 as tall, clear, and bright.

You see a shop window, above which hangs a sign saying "Ladies' Happiness."

Breathe out. In the shop window, see your child, radiant as a saint enthroned among beautiful treasures from all parts of the world.

Breathe out. Open your eyes, seeing your radiant child with open eyes.

QUICKENING

You have waited to know if you were pregnant, waited for your first trimester to end so you will feel better. Now you wait for the first signs of what is called "quickening," a beautiful word meaning to stir, to stimulate, to show signs of life. The quickening is a milestone in your pregnancy. For me, that first fluttering came as a great surprise. I cried out and laughed. It felt so weird and so good to sense him moving within, as if someone were caressing or tickling the inside of my belly. I called him my little fish.

You will begin to feel these movements somewhere between your 16th and 22nd weeks when your baby is big enough to reach out and touch the boundaries of his uterine home. Don't worry if you don't feel anything by the 16th week; you have time. Your child is moving in your womb even if you don't feel him yet, and the first perceptible move-ments can be very slight and subtle. One day as he stirs, your uterine muscles will feel stimulated. You may experience these fetal movements as a fluttering sensation in the lower abdomen or as a light tapping. Later, as your baby gets bigger, his acrobatics will feel more like kicks.

When you experience that strange fluttering for the first time, the sensation will surprise you and fill you with joy. Your baby is alive! Even though you've seen him moving on the monitor screen, it is a profound *aha!* when you actually feel him for the first time. You will want to bring your partner's hand to your belly to feel this miracle.

After that, of course, you will be monitoring every movement your baby makes and wondering when was the last time you felt him move. Don't get obsessive about this. In the beginning it may happen only every other day. As your baby gets bigger, you will feel his move-ments more frequently, though you may not notice them if you're too busy or if you're sleeping. Eventually you will even be able to *see* your baby moving by looking at your belly. Babies are often very active at night. Following is an exercise to help quiet you and quicken your baby.

⋰⋱

WHITE PETALS
exercise 44

Close your eyes. Breathe out slowly three times, counting from 3 to 1, seeing the numbers in your mind's eye. See the number 1 as tall, clear, and bright.

Imagine you are in a field full of white flowers. Gather a big bouquet of them. Lie down in the tall grass next to a running brook.

Breathe out. Pluck the white petals from the flowers and cover your abdomen with them. Feel the sap and the life force that permeate the petals entering your womb.

Breathe out. Sense and see the petals absorbing all that is not absolutely perfect for you and your child.

Breathe out. Once the petals have turned brown from absorbing what is not absolutely perfect, gather them up from your abdomen and throw them into the nearby brook.

Breathe out. Do it again and again until the petals you put on your abdomen remain white.

Breathe out. Rest, sensing your child stirring within you. See and feel the dome of the sky covering you and your unborn child with its protective blue aura.

Breathe out. Open your eyes, feeling refreshed.

Baby's movements are his form of communication. He will tap or kick if he is frightened or upset but also when he is stimulated. As soon as you can identify your baby's movements in the womb, begin communicating by responding to his tap with a caress, or tap at the same place on your abdomen. You can also try tapping to see if your baby answers back. Do so rhythmically and at set intervals, like Morse code. What a delight when he answers back! But don't overdo it. Your baby needs to sleep for long stretches of time and mustn't be interrupted. You will soon learn to recognize when he is awake by his movements. Like you, he has clear patterns of waking and sleep, which are unique to him, so don't go worrying about whether he has the "right" pattern. He does. Caress him to reassure him. Tap to communicate, and as a way of playing with your unborn child.

RESTING AND IMMERSION

As you grow rounder with your pregnancy, both your body and your baby need more of your attention. It is a matter of resting with attentiveness. Do this easily, without effort. Hypervigilance is contraindicated. Learn to hover over the unfolding new world you have generated. Sit and dream like a brooding hen or a bird in her nest, in sympathetic communication with your progeny.

In your dreaming, you will become one with your dreaming baby. The word "dream" in Hebrew, *chalom,* has the same root as the sweet, braided bread that is customarily served for shabbath, called *chala.* This suggests that your dreaming is an important ingredient in the rising and taste of that sacred bread. In the same way, your dreamy attentiveness and loving-kindness play a major part in the "cooking" of your unborn child. Whatever you are busy with, never cease to shower your unborn child with mindfulness and love to greatly enhance your mutual interchange and bonding.

SECRET GARDEN
exercise 45

Close your eyes. Breathe out slowly three times, counting from 3 to 1, seeing the numbers in your mind's eye. See the number 1 as tall, clear, and bright.

Imagine that you are standing in front of a circular walled garden. Walk around the walls until you find the gate. Find the key to the gate and unlock the gate.

Breathe out. Walk into the garden. What does it look like? Are there flowers? What colors? How do they smell?

Breathe out. If the garden needs tending, do so until the garden looks just as you want it to look.

Breathe out. Walk deeper into the garden, toward the center. Find a beautiful, strong tree that offers shade and sit in its shade on a patch of thick, emerald-green grass.

Breathe out. Listen for water nearby. Hear the sounds of nature. Feel yourself breathing with nature, in rhythm with its cycles.

Breathe out. Feel and see your baby responding to your breathing as he also becomes attuned to the rhythms of nature.

Breathe out. Rest and relax, enjoying nature and your baby until you feel rejuvenated.

Breathe out. Get up and walk back out of your garden, your baby safely tucked under your heart. Notice whether anything looks different as you go.

Breathe out. Close the gate behind you and lock it, taking the key or hiding it in some safe place where you can find it whenever you need it.

Breathe out. Open your eyes, asking that the feeling of rest and peacefulness continue for both of you throughout your day.

Allowing yourself to rest is *not* an indulgence. It is a necessity. Both you and your child need it. Your body needs to concentrate all its energies on keeping you healthy while feeding the growing life within your womb. Your baby is growing, and he needs your physical and mental energies. As you now know, your mental energies are as important to your baby's development as are your physical energies. Try to rest at least once a day, every day, at lunchtime. Take a half hour's rest, lying down if possible, emptying your mind, and visiting your child. You can incorporate the *Secret garden* (page 95) and *Going into the womb to visit your child* (page 66) exercises. While the exercises are very short, a maximum of three to five minutes, you will feel as if you have taken a very long rest. Rest comes from allowing for the dreamtime. Doing it consciously during the day, as well as subconsciously at night, brings inestimable benefits to both you and your baby.

WHO IS MY CHILD?

When you allow yourself rest and immersion in your pregnancy, your "knowing" of your child develops on a wordless, subconscious level. You "know" the unfolding of his nervous system, brain, and skin; you sense that his organs are beginning to take on their individualized tasks. Your child's incarnation in a physical body is becoming more and more real and defined. While your right brain basks in the experience, your left brain asks questions, since this is its nature: Who is this child? Will I like him? Will we get along? I know that I had those questions during my pregnancy. I toyed with the mystery as one turns round and round in one's hands an unopened Christmas gift. I held on to my questions to prolong the fearful anticipation and joy. Every day I prayed: make us compatible; make us like and understand each other.

The question of naming came up in our family, as it will around this time in yours. What are we going to call this bundle of mystery? The quest for a name focuses all our tormenting questions. A name is meaningful. Many ancient traditions believe that the given name holds a powerful vibratory truth. It both circumscribes and impacts the personality and goals of the one who carries it. My stepchildren wanted to call my son Zack. I "knew" he wasn't a Zack. It was too nervous a name, too zigzaggy, like the lightning bolts in our sky that summer. I asked my dreams: What is he like? What is his name?

> I see a crib with wooden bars. An infant stands in the crib
> holding a snake in each hand and squeezing them to death.
> I hear a voice loudly calling out, "My name is Sam!"

If you were brought up like me, in the knowledge of Greek myths, you will immediately recognize the boy in the crib who kills the two snakes. He is young Hercules, who later becomes the strong man of Greek mythology. He has a tall, powerful physique.

The dream was clairvoyant in two undeniable and powerful ways. Both Sam's paternal great-grandfathers, long dead, were called Sam, though I didn't know it at the time. It is the religious custom in Jewish families to name the child after a dead ancestor. As for Sam (yes, we listened to the dream and named him Sam!), he has turned out to be a great hulk of a man with a powerful presence. He is now twenty-six

97

years old. We have a natural intimacy and understanding of each other, which I attribute to my prayers.

Some mothers look at their child and see a stranger. They don't know what makes him tick. This is very sad. Start now to get to "know" your child. Learn by osmosis. Dream with him, and you will weave a tapestry of splendid colors and scenes together.

⚜

WEAVING YOUR CHILD'S LIFE TAPESTRY AND NAME
exercise 46

Close your eyes. Breathe out slowly three times, counting from 3 to 1, seeing the numbers in your mind's eye. See the number 1 as tall, clear, and bright.

Imagine you are sitting in front of your loom. In your lap, you have many skeins of colored wool.

Breathe out. Turn your eyes inward to contact your child. Ask him what color you should use. See the color that pops up for you, and start weaving.

Breathe out. Each time you change color, check with your child and see which color pops up.

Breathe out. When you feel that your tapestry is done, look at the scene you have woven.

Breathe out. If you feel something needs to be changed, do so. Do this until you are satisfied.

Breathe out. Turn your eyes inward and check with your child that the tapestry of his life is to his liking.

Breathe out. Ask his name. If you feel satisfied with it, weave it into the tapestry.

Breathe out. Open your eyes, seeing the tapestry with open eyes and hearing his name.

BODY CHANGES AND CHALLENGES

Pregnancy is about accepting gratefully and graciously that your body is changing. Each sign of change is evidence that your baby is growing and that your body is adjusting to more of your baby's presence. This can prove stressful, and your body may need some help adjusting. As Chinese medicine points out, it is the nature of human physicality that every one of us lives with some form of imbalance. We either have too little of something or too much: too much fire and not enough earth, or too much air and no water. Rebalancing your body is important to the healthy continuation of your pregnancy. Often a short exercise is all you need to help your body readjust.

Anemia, high blood pressure, edema, backache, leg cramps, numbness in the fingers, breathlessness, and sleep disturbances are some of the issues that may occur. We will deal with each of these mostly minor stresses one by one. More serious challenges, such as placenta previa or premature contractions, are rare. You will find the necessary exercises for these issues in appendix 2 (page 291).

Anemia

In the second trimester, especially after the 20th week, blood volume increases as your baby grows. You will need more iron to produce red blood cells. Your doctor will prescribe an iron supplement and suggest iron-rich foods, such as artichokes or potatoes including the skin. But your iron stores may already be depleted by poor nutrition, heavy morning sickness, successive pregnancies, or carrying twins. Symptoms of anemia include extreme fatigue, weakness, pallor, palpitations, and fainting spells.

If you have those symptoms or if you want simply to boost your blood counts and overall energy, practice the following exercises called the *Blue vase*. It is best to do this exercise in the morning. You do not want to boost your energy at night when you are about to go to sleep. Practice this exercise for a maximum of three minutes, not longer.

BLUE VASE
exercise 47

Find a quiet place where you are not likely to be disturbed and where you can relax. Sit in an armchair with your arms and legs uncrossed. Close your eyes.

Breathe out all that disturbs you, all that tires you, all that obscures you.

Breathe it out as a light smoke that is easily absorbed by the plant life around you.

When your breath comes in on the inhalation, see it as blue and filled with sunlight, like the radiant blue light from the sky.

See the blue-gold light filling your nostrils, your mouth, your throat, and flowing down your back like a great river of light. See it filling your legs, your feet and your toes, and stretching out of your toes as long antennas of light.

See the light circulating up your legs to fill your pelvis.

See the clear blue light surrounding and cushioning the amniotic sac in which your baby is floating comfortably. See the light rising up into your chest, filling your breasts, and radiating out of them.

See it flowing in and out of your heart until your heart becomes a glowing blue lamp.

See the light flow down your arms like smaller rivers of light, filling your hands and fingers, stretching out of your fingers as long antennae of light.

As you continue to breathe in the blue light, see the light continue to fill you.

See it begin to radiate out of the articulations of your joints, out of your ankles, knees, hips, shoulders, elbows, and wrists.

See the light fill you until it radiates out of your skin in all directions.

See yourself as a crystal vase filled with light, the light cushioning the globe of blue amniotic waters in which your baby floats. See yourself radiating light in all directions.

Breathe out, open your eyes, and see this with open eyes for a few seconds.

Practice this exercise for twenty-one days, stop for seven, and then practice for another twenty-one days. Soon the subconscious will be doing the exercise for you; you will not need to do it so consistently. From time to time, you can do it to give yourself a reminder or a boost.

High Blood Pressure

Blood pressure varies throughout your pregnancy. From your baseline reading at the beginning of your pregnancy, it drops a little and then rises again around the seventh month. Stress, anxiety, or simply being rushed can affect your readings. This is nothing to worry about. Worry will only make the readings go up. Practice your *Natural breathing* exercise (page 41). It will help you to relax. Your doctor will tell you if your blood pressure is too high. He will need at least two readings to determine that.

Meanwhile, if you are worried about your blood pressure reading, here's a good exercise to prove to yourself that you are the mind behind your body. Do *not* do this exercise if you don't have blood pressure issues.

WHITE STAIRCASE
exercise 48

Close your eyes. Breathe out slowly three times, counting from 3 to 1, seeing the numbers in your mind's eye. See the number 1 as tall, clear, and bright.

Imagine that you are standing at the foot of a large white marble staircase. Start climbing up. As you go up, your clothes are progressively getting lighter in color until they turn completely white when you reach the top of the staircase.

Breathe out. Now turn around and come down the staircase dressed all in white. Step off the staircase dressed in white.

Breathe out. Open your eyes, seeing yourself wearing all white.

Now ask the nurse to check your blood pressure again.

Anyone with chronic hypertension should do this exercise three times a day or more if needed. Do it for twenty-one days, stop for three days, and start again. As you learn to produce better images for your subconscious to work with, you will also need to modify your diet, drink a lot of fluids, and get plenty of rest and relaxation.

Edema

Swelling of your hands and feet is a side effect of carrying your baby. Your body is not always strong enough to deal with an added load that is getting heavier every day. Get off your feet, rest more, or take a brisk walk for a few minutes to increase circulation. Swelling is connected to waste products accumulating in your system. Increasing your fluid intake will help flush them out. So will the following exercise.

THE RIVER RUNS THROUGH
exercise 49

Close your eyes. Breathe out slowly three times, counting from 3 to 1, seeing the numbers in your mind's eye. See the number 1 as tall, clear, and bright.

Imagine walking in a sunny meadow. Hear the sound of water. Walk toward it.

Breathe out. Look down at the clear mountain brook and its sandy bottom. Take off your clothes, and, telling Baby that you are going to step into the brook, lie down on the sandy bottom, head toward the mountain, feet toward the ocean.

Breathe out. Feel the water washing you from head to foot, caressing your breasts, your belly, your legs, opening up the pores of your skin.

Breathe out. Now your pores are wide open. The river begins to flow through your body, around the amniotic sac, down through your legs and out your toes and the soles of your feet, washing away any waste products that are clogging your body. Stay there until your body becomes translucent and you can see your baby floating quietly in his own amniotic waters.

Breathe out. Step out of the water and stretch yourself in the sunlight. Sing and dance until you are dry.

Breathe out. Returning to your clothes, see that your old clothes are gone and that new pastel or white loose clothing is awaiting you. Put it on, feeling the soft texture caressing your bare skin and belly. Caress your baby through the cloth, feeling refreshed and happy.

Breathe out. Open your eyes, seeing yourself wearing your new clothes, your feet and hands trim and pliant, your baby comfortably tucked under your heart.

This exercise will help reduce your swelling, and you can also use it if you ate or drank something that didn't agree with you. You should feel an immediate alleviation of your symptoms.

Even if you feel better after doing the exercise, see your doctor right away if your swelling is accompanied by a sudden weight gain and increase in blood pressure, as you may be showing the first symptoms of preeclampsia. Since preeclampsia (also called toxemia) is a high blood pressure–related condition, don't forget to practice the *White staircase* (page 102) every hour on the hour for three days, then three or more times a day for twenty-one days. If the word "preeclampsia" frightens you, remember that you are not a victim of your diagnosis, nor are you totally dependent on outside help. You can do mind exercises to better your situation.

Follow your doctor's advice, of course, but also use your "mind over matter" tools. Your imagination is the powerhouse behind your immune system. The exercises in this book are crafted precisely to engineer the specific changes you are seeking. Practice them and make a note of your results. The more you exercise the muscles of your imagination, the better your results will be.

Backache, Leg Cramps, Numbness in the Fingers, Tingling in the Extremities, Breathlessness

Why am I lumping all these symptoms together? Can one exercise help relieve them all? Think of the load you are carrying. Your baby is getting heavier by the minute. You can't put him down. You can only put yourself in a prone position. By taking the weight off your spine, you relieve your back pain for a moment. But does it relieve your leg cramps, the numbness in your fingers, the tingling in your extremities, your breathlessness?

Swelling that is pressing down on nerves is thought to be one of the causes of numbness in the fingers and tingling in the extremities. It can also be a factor in leg cramps. You know what to do for swelling. *The river runs through* exercise (page 103) will help.

But ultimately, the key factor in all these different symptoms is the health of your spine. Your spine is made up of separate components—vertebrae—cushioned by a cartilage mass called intervertebral discs that act as shock absorbers. They compress when you're lifting weights and spring back when you're at rest. Nerves branch out of your spine toward major organs and limbs. Numbness or tingling results from compressed discs pinching the nerves.

Every pregnancy book will stress the importance of exercise. Aerobics (not too strenuous), calisthenics, weight training, and yoga are all excellent choices when tailored to the needs of the pregnant woman. But what most training systems fail to tell you is that imagery—the language the subconscious mind understands and accepts as its command cue—physically exercises your body by activating micromovements in your muscles.

MICROMOVEMENTS
exercise 50

Close your eyes. Breathe out slowly three times, counting from 3 to 1. See the 1 as tall, clear, and bright.

See yourself running. Have all the appropriate sensations. What is happening in your calf muscles?

Breathe out. Open your eyes.

If you pay attention, you will feel your calf muscles microcontracting. Micromovement is what really trains your body. Using mind over matter will allow you to pump up your muscles much faster than plain exercise without visualizations. Olympic athletes are taught to visualize their jumps or ski runs. Every mom going into labor is an Olympic athlete in training. The word "labor" itself strongly suggests the need to get in shape. You will more easily meet your athletic challenge by practicing your imagery. I will be giving you precise imagery exercises to train for "labor."

Next is the first of the exercises that will help get you into good physical shape. Do this to elongate your spine, keep your discs from compressing, and teach yourself better posture. Do the exercise without moving. Let the images move your body. If you have any pain, stop.

ALICE IN WONDERLAND
exercise 51

Close your eyes. Breathe out slowly three times, counting from 3 to 1, seeing the numbers in your mind's eye. See the number 1 as tall, clear, and bright.

Sense, see, and feel that like Alice in Wonderland, you are stretching your neck up and up until your head touches the ceiling.

Breathe out. Look down. What do your arms and legs look like? Are they longer, shorter, or the same size as before? If they are not long, then grow them. See your feet grow down through the floor and down into the earth. See your arms stretch through the floor and your fingers reach down into the earth below.

Breathe out. Now extend your head up through the ceiling, then through the roof up into the sky. Look over the rooftop.

Breathe out. Turn your head slowly to look over your right shoulder and beyond. Do not strain yourself. Gaze over the rooftops.

Breathe out. Now bring your head slowly forward. Turn your head slowly to look over your left shoulder and beyond. Bring it back forward.

Breathe out. Look up at the sky; now bring the back of your head to touch your spine. Bring it forward again.

Breathe out. Now roll your head down into your chest. Bring it back.

Breathe out. Bring yourself back down through the roof, returning to your normal size. Return your arms and legs to their normal size at the same time.

Breathe out. Now ask your body to add an inch, in a single block or in sections, to any part(s) of your body it wants. See where the elongation occurs.

Breathe out. Sense this with open eyes.

Here is a simpler form of the exercise.

NUMBER 1

exercise 52

Close your eyes. Breathe out slowly three times, counting from 3 to 1, seeing the numbers in your mind's eye. See the number 1 as tall, clear, and bright—like a tall, bright column.

Step into the 1. Feel your body becoming one with the tall, bright column. Sense how the bulge of your belly is supported by the elongated spine.

Breathe out. Open your eyes, sensing and seeing the elongation with open eyes.

Elongating your cervical vertebrae frees the nerves that travel down to your fingertips. Elongating your lumbar vertebrae frees the nerves to your legs and feet. When your nerves are free, the tingling at your extremities disappears. Elongation also restores space to your rib cage. Releasing your lungs and diaphragm helps relieve your breathlessness.

Remember: Visualize your movement before physically moving. Have all the sensations of the movement when you're visualizing. It will greatly enhance any physical program you're engaged in.

Sleep Disturbances

Sleep has never been a problem for you, but suddenly you are having a hard time settling down at night. You wake up to go to the bathroom and can't get back to sleep. You have trouble finding a position that feels comfortable. You toss and turn. Your baby kicks. You worry about a new mouth to feed, about how your partner will adapt to the new baby, about what will happen with your job. Your skin feels stretched, your belly itches, your hemorrhoids hurt, your baby is dancing a jig, you're having a hard time digesting your meal, and you need to pee again!

Don't eat and go straight to bed. Give yourself time to digest. Don't sleep on your stomach or back. Sleep on your side, a large soft pillow between your legs. That will help a little. But what is more important is quieting your mind. Do the following exercises in bed.

OCEAN OF LIGHT (1)
exercise 53

Close your eyes. Breathe out slowly three times, counting from 3 to 1, seeing the numbers in your mind's eye. See the number 1 as tall, clear, and bright.

Imagine that you are walking near the ocean on a warm, star-studded night. The moon is full and illuminates the ocean with moonlight.

Breathe out. Imagine that you lie down on the ocean of light. Feel it cushioning you and your baby. Feel your body relaxing limb by limb, your neck and head sinking into the soft, cushiony moonlight. Feel the light enveloping and supporting you.

Breathe out. Listen to the symphony of the stars as they sing you to sleep.

There are other ways to quiet the mind. Do the following exercise after you have finished the *Ocean of light* exercise if you are still awake. You will be feeling very relaxed. Review your day, moving backward from the present. As you watch, allow what you see to sink in without judgment or commentary, simply recognizing it for what it is.

REVERSING
exercise 54

Begin looking at your day, moving backward from the present.
Just before turning off the light, you were reading a book.
See yourself doing that, acknowledging all the thought forms
that came along with your reading. Before going to bed, you
brushed your teeth. Rewind the tape: going to bed, leaving
the bathroom, brushing your teeth. Recognize the sensations
and thought forms that came with brushing your teeth. Move
back through your day's activities one by one, noting what
happened and what you felt each time. If there is a difficult
moment with someone, breathe out and reassure your baby
that you and he are fine and there is nothing for him to worry
about. Then imagine that you step into the shoes of the person
you are confronting, taking his or her exact position. You'll
now get a view of yourself as he or she sees you. At this
moment, he or she serves as your dreaming mirror. You will
see, from his or her viewpoint, how you looked, how you
moved, how you behaved, and how you sounded to him or her
when you had the confrontation. Return to your own place;
look at that person with new eyes. Continue reversing. Do so
until you fall asleep or reach the morning of your reversed day.

Most people will fall asleep long before they have gone all the way
back to the morning in their reversing. This exercise is also called
Exam of conscience backward. If you do it regularly each night, you
will clear the day's events and be able to begin the next day with a
fresh view of things. You will sleep better and have more energy for
the next day.

SUPPORT

The stresses I've been speaking of are usually only skin deep. Like mosquito bites on a summer's day at the beach, they cannot spoil your happiness. Your second trimester is one of joyful expectation laced with occasional mild apprehension. It is a time when you will be thinking of choosing between a hospital and a home birth, shopping around for childbirth classes, and deciding whether to have a doula (a labor coach who also offers prenatal and postpartum support). You will be exploring what kind of birth you want and when you will feel the need for female advice and support. You may already have such support among family members and friends who have already given birth.

You may not have such support, however. I didn't, as I was new to this country. My mother was in France, my teacher in Israel. While I had my husband, a compassionate doctor willing to listen to all my concerns, I didn't realize how bereft I was of women's company until I was taking a walk in the woods with writer Annie Dillard. I must have voiced my longing because the next day she invited me to a restaurant where she had gathered twenty of her women friends to speak to me about their birthing experiences! One of them had had eight children. "Childbirth is the greatest orgasm you'll ever have!" Nancy Watson, a children's book author, told me. She knew, for her eight children had been born through natural childbirth. She and Annie are part of the reason I am writing this book—to thank those generous friends for gifting me with such abundance and laughter!

Remember, there are women all around you who are already mothers. Talk to them, but choose your friends carefully. Don't listen to the doomsday gossips. What they say will affect you, even against your will. Choose friends who have a positive, healthy outlook on life!

One way to tap into support is by connecting with your ancestors. Your roots are always with you. Even if you don't know who your birth mother or your grandmother were, you still have roots. They are embedded in the fact that no one is born without a mother. You are part of a great chain of mothers. You are a living tree of life, your long lineage stretching back into the past in one great, unbroken line. You, in turn, are participating in this amazing chain of events, as you hover over your unborn child and prepare to bring him forth into the world.

ANCESTRY SUPPORT
exercise 55

Close your eyes. Breathe out slowly three times, counting from 3 to 1, seeing the numbers in your mind's eye. See the number 1 as tall, clear, and bright.

See the women around you who are positive and supportive. See their faces. How many are there?

Breathe out. Behind your women friends, see your female ancestors all the way back to Eve.

Breathe out. Have them surround you and hold you from behind.

Sense and know that the Divine Mother is behind all of them, supporting them in supporting you. Sink back into their arms and let yourself be held.

Breathe out. Open your eyes, feeling their support with open eyes.

TREE OF LIFE
exercise 56

Close your eyes. Breathe out slowly three times, counting from 3 to 1, seeing the numbers in your mind's eye. See the number 1 as tall, clear, and bright.

See yourself as a tree of life that is enveloping you and your baby in a luminous green aura. Bask together in that luminous aura, enjoying the verdant serenity of creation.

Breathe out. Open your eyes, feeling the serenity with open eyes.

As you approach the end of the second trimester, you can look back on a road well traveled. You have taken good care of yourself and of your baby. Through your mind exercises, you have enjoyed the serenity of your brooding period. You have rested, contemplated, and dreamed. Like a good long-distance runner, you are entering the last lap of the race ahead of the game. You have set the pace, and you are ready for the final spurt that will take you to the finish line.

5

The Rush to Prepare

Before I formed thee in the belly I knew thee; and
before thou camest forth out of the womb.

JEREMIAH 1:5

IN THE FINAL stretch before you give birth, the symbiosis between you and your child is reaching perfection. In this last trimester, your body is preparing, like a skin, to burst open and let forth the "fruit of your womb." Soon the fruit will become too weighty to support. It will drop, beginning its climactic journey toward individuation. At this moment, you are both blooming and untouchable, like Mary, mother and virgin, who carries the god within. Like hers, your child is divine, by virtue of this mysterious unfolding that is reaching maturity in your depths. You are the creation goddess, exhausted by the final climb up the mountain, exuberant at seeing the summit above. Your moods oscillate between lethargy and intense busyness. You probably can't quite put it into words, but ever present in you is this expectation of the great advent of your child. As the fruit of your womb grows ever fuller, you are put on notice that it is no longer time to be idle but to come down to earth and ground yourself in preparations for your child's arrival.

BECOMING A MOM

You have known for six months that you're going to be a mom, but now the realization takes on a different meaning. You are in countdown mode. Your due date is no longer far in the nebulous future. You are committed, and there's no turning back. It's time to bring your dreams into reality, time to prepare your nest for the new arrival.

You may have been preparing for just this time and are now joyously expectant. In fact, like a mama bird, you will find yourself becoming increasingly busy, actively rearranging your home, ordering the crib, and choosing colors for the walls. You will be going far afield to gather all the items you need to take care of your child once she arrives. Your concrete preparations will keep you occupied and take the edge off both your excitement and your exhaustion at having to wait just a little while longer.

The task of concretely preparing for your child's arrival could bring forth untold fears. Suddenly you're confronted with the looming reality of a completely vulnerable being who will be entirely dependent on you. Don't start comparing yourself with the other moms-to-be who are looking, as far as you can see, so very complacent and satisfied. Even they have fearful moments. Your idea that they're going to be perfect moms is just as far-fetched as your fear that you most certainly won't be. Once your child is born, you may find that the very natural, innate knowing that just shows up for us mothers, if we listen to it, will be there for you. You simply know what to do.

What are the fears that come up at this point? Fear of commitment, fear of not being a good mom, fear of being just like your own mother, fear of physical closeness. It is good to deal with these before your child is born so that when your child arrives, there is no emotional baggage blocking the way.

Fear of Commitment

Having to be responsible for a completely vulnerable being can be quite overwhelming. The time commitment and emotional involvement are not to be underestimated. You may be used to working outside the home in a competitive career. You are used to having your own creative and self-empowering activities. The thought of giving up your ambitions to become a nursemaid may upset you. And that is perfectly legitimate! You don't necessarily want to be the housewife and mom your own mother was. In the words of writer and anthropologist Mary Catherine Bateson, you will have to learn to "compose a life" for yourself that will encompass your different interests. At this time, however, as you begin giving serious thought to how to manage a career, a relationship, a new baby, and older kids if you have them, you may feel resentful and protective of your own time. You may be thinking, *What about me?* How can you deal with your own sense of panic over what is about to befall you?

Fear of Not Being a Good Mom

What makes you think you won't be a good mom? Maybe your sibling was always considered more able and mature than you. Maybe you were told you would never make a good mom because you weren't nurturing. Maybe you feel that you have never grown up and still need a lot of nurturing yourself.

❧

FREEING THE INNER CHILD
exercise 57

Close your eyes. Breathe out slowly three times, counting from 3 to 1, seeing the numbers in your mind's eye. See the number 1 as tall, clear, and bright.

Tell your child that you are going to do an exercise now, that whatever emotions you feel should not concern her, and that all is well and she is safe in her amniotic sac, tucked comfortably under your heart.

See the child in you. Where is she? What is she doing? Take care of whatever necessity appears. For instance, if the child is in a corner crying, do what is necessary to console her.

Breathe out. Take the child out into a meadow to run and play. Play with her. Tell her she is now free to have fun, and that you will play with her.

Breathe out and open your eyes.

You have retrieved some part of yourself that you had lost. You can now be more present when your child comes. Remember that your child wants you as a mother, whatever your mothering style. It is your smell, your voice that she gravitates toward, not anyone else's. You are the mother she wants. She is yours unless you drive her away.

Fear of Being Like Mom

But what if you are afraid of being just like your mom? Whether for good or for bad, we learn through imitation. Even though you may not like the way your mother was as a mom, you have learned her ways; they are part of your subconscious baggage. What if you were to act as she did? What if you turn out to be an angry, violent, rejecting, or absent mother just like her? This is a very real fear. *Freeing the inner child* (page 117) helped you face yourself as a mother, and the exercise *Taking your mother out of your body* (page 120) you will help you face your own mother.

REVERSING THE PAST
exercise 58

Close your eyes. Breathe out slowly three times, counting from 3 to 1, seeing the numbers in your mind's eye. See the number 1 as tall, clear, and bright.

Tell your child that you are going to do an exercise now, that whatever emotions you feel should not concern her, and that all is well and she is safe in her amniotic sac, tucked comfortably under your heart.

Go back to the very first time you ever felt difficulty with your mother. See where you are, what is happening, and how old you are.

Breathe out. Imagine that you, the adult, move to stand next to yourself as a child. Tell her you are protecting her now, and she can express what she feels to her mother. She must do so in the child's voice.

Breathe out. Tell her that you are going to cut the negative cord between her and her mother. Now cut the cord. What happens? If her mother fades away, you have cut the right cord. If not, know there is another invisible cord that needs to be cut. This time, cut it with a sword. See her mother fading away.

Breathe out. Take the child out into a meadow to run and play. Play with her. Tell her she is now free to grow up.

Breathe out. See the child beginning to grow before your eyes through all the stages of childhood, adolescence, and young adulthood until you are both the same height and standing face to face.

Breathe out. Look into the eyes of this other you and embrace her. See and live what happens when you embrace.

Breathe out. Feel her merging into you, and be grateful that this lost part of you has returned to you.

Breathe out and open your eyes.

Having faced your mother and cut the negative cord, you have freed yourself from those emotionally difficult memories. Now you must take your mother out of your body: not your love for her (this you must keep) but her physicality. If she remains there, you might be driven to imitate her words and gestures. The subconscious is programmed by the sound, smell, taste, touch, and sight of events that are emotionally traumatic. If the way your mother behaved toward you resulted in emotional trauma, you are imprinted with her ways. You have just cut the cord. Now here's how to take her out of your body and your subconscious. Remember that the mother you are taking out of your body today may be only one aspect of the total mother experience you are holding. You can repeat this exercise as many times as you feel you need to.

TAKING YOUR MOTHER OUT OF YOUR BODY
exercise 59

Close your eyes. Breathe out slowly three times, counting from 3 to 1, seeing the numbers in your mind's eye. See the number 1 as tall, clear, and bright.

Tell your child that you are going to do an exercise now, that whatever emotions you feel should not concern her, and that all is well and she is safe in her amniotic sac, tucked comfortably under your heart.

Turn your eyes inward and find where your mother is lodged in your body. Tell her that you are now an adult and that having her in your body is no longer appropriate. Politely ask her to leave.

Breathe out. If she won't go, lift your hands up toward the sun, stretching your arms until your hands are close to the sun. Feel them getting warm and turning into light. Bring your hands down into your body. Take your mother by the shoulders and take her out of your body. Place her to the right or to the left of you, as you see fit.

Breathe out. Pour cool, clear spring water into the spaces vacated by your mother. Ask every cell in your body to return to its natural, healthy alignment.

Breathe out and open your eyes, feeling free and whole.

By taking your mother out of your body, you have decided you will no longer be the victim of your past. You have become responsible for yourself, which means that you choose response over reactivity. This will make it easier for you to become the parent you dream of being: fair and loving and able to cope calmly with your child's moods. For, as you know, little kids are very reactive and emotional. Being able to handle and regulate your own emotions will make it easier for you to teach your children how to regulate theirs.

Fear of physical closeness with those you most want to be close to often comes from having been hurt or abused as a child. Letting go of old fears can be done simply and easily without having to refer back to those old pains. You don't need to look into the garbage bag when you throw out the trash.

THE CYLINDRICAL MIRROR
exercise 60

Close your eyes. Breathe out slowly three times, counting from 3 to 1, seeing the numbers in your mind's eye. See the number 1 as tall, clear, and bright.

Tell your child that you are going to do an exercise now, that whatever emotions you feel should not concern her, and that all is well and she is safe in her amniotic sac, tucked comfortably under your heart.

Imagine that you are standing in front of a mirrored column that is slowly turning. Watch as from every recess or fold of your body memories rise up like smoke. You don't need to know what those memories are. Just see them as smoke. When the mirrored column stops turning, you have let go of the memories your body is ready to let go of today.

Breathe out. See yourself in the mirrored column, free of those memories you no longer need. What do you look like now?

Breathe out. Open your eyes, feeling lighter and refreshed.

Fear of physical closeness can also come from your physical type. If you have a nervous body with little flesh on it, you may not be the cuddly type. Pregnancy will help by fleshing you out. And that is a good thing, as babies need a lot of cuddling and skin-to-skin contact with their mothers, especially in the beginning (see chapter 7; you will find exercises there to help you bond with your baby). In either case, whether it is because of your type or because of hurt or abuse, do the following exercise to give yourself some tender loving care. Think of it as a self-healing exercise.

TLC FOR YOURSELF
exercise 61

Close your eyes. Breathe out slowly three times, counting from 3 to 1, seeing the numbers in your mind's eye. See the number 1 as tall, clear, and bright.

Imagine that you are in a meadow on a bright, sunny day. Lift your arms up toward the sun and feel them elongating until your hands are close to the sun. Feel them getting warmer, turning into light.

Breathe out. Bring your arms down, keeping them a few inches away from your body, and sweep your hands, palms toward you, up from your feet to your face, then over your head and down your back. Since your arms are long, this is easy to do.

Breathe out. Imagine that you pass your hands under the soles of your feet and up the front of your body again. Do this three times, feeling the warmth and the light sweeping your body.

Breathe out. Imagine that you lie down in the green grass. Hold your hands a few inches away from your hips. Feel the warmth and the light of your hands, and feel your hips and legs relaxing. Accept whatever sensations arise. If memories arise, let them go like smoke rising out of your body.

Breathe out. Place your two hands at the height of your breasts, a few inches away. Feel the warmth and the light of your hands. Accept whatever sensations arise. If memories arise, let them go like smoke rising out of your body.

Breathe out. Open your eyes.

Do not push yourself. Go slowly. You can repeat this exercise once a day. You will have less fear of your child's body when you start loving your own body. Many of these exercises will help you reclaim your body with all its sensations, pleasures, and pains. This takes courage. Congratulations! Reclaiming your body helps you be more fully present to yourself and to your child.

PREPARING FOR LABOR

As I have said, parenting starts long before the actual birth of your child. Preparing your birth experience is part of parenting. Both you and your child are on the verge of an extraordinary burst of activity that will bring this phase of your adventure together to an end. That it is called labor suggests that much physical and mental exertion are involved. It makes sense to prepare yourself, as Olympic athletes do, by visually rehearsing all the steps that will lead you toward a triumphant outcome.

As you know, images are the language of your body. When you visualize with precision what you want to obtain from your body, you are actually sending orders that your body responds to in micro-movements. You are doing your warm-up exercises. You are helping your body by letting it know what actually needs to happen now.

Start rehearsing the birth in the 32nd week (beginning of the eighth month) or, if you're carrying twins, in the 28th week. You will be doing this exercise every day once a day (or more, if you wish) until the baby's birth. Do it during your lunch break, when you can take time to rest and reconnect with your baby—and do it only after you have made contact with your baby using *Going into the womb to visit your child* (page 66). You will find a modified version incorporated in the following script that is your main exercise for rehearsing the birth.

REHEARSING THE BIRTH—THE FLOWER
exercise 62

Close your eyes. Breathe out slowly three times, counting from 3 to 1, seeing the numbers in your mind's eye. See the number 1 as tall, clear, and bright.

Turn your eyes inward into your body. Your eyes are very bright, illuminating the way. Travel down to the amniotic sac.

Breathe out. When you come to it, look in to see your baby floating freely and comfortably in the clear blue amniotic waters.

Breathe out. Make eye contact with your baby, smile, and talk to her, telling her everything you want to say today.

Breathe out. Tell your baby that you and she are going to rehearse her birth. You are going to show her exactly what will happen when she is ready to be born. Tell her how excited you are at the thought of soon seeing her face and holding her in your arms. You are going to lead your baby through a visualization of her perfect birth.

Breathe out. Visualize your baby turning to be head down, face toward your sacrum, in the perfect birthing position. See that the cord is floating upward from the belly button, free and unencumbered, and will remain so throughout the birth.

Breathe out. See that your baby's head is resting at the stem of an upside-down flower whose bud is beginning to open up slowly, petal by petal, until the flower is completely and widely open.

Breathe out. Now visualize your baby sliding down the stem of the flower in a rush of waters and lubricating oils, the cord floating up freely.

Breathe out. See your baby come out through the wide opening of the flower into a magnificent garden and into your partner's arms.

Breathe out. See your partner placing your baby on your chest. Feel the exhilaration and joy as you hold her in your arms and look at her face for the first time. Hear all of nature rejoicing in the arrival of your newborn.

Breathe out and open your eyes.

While we have no clinical trials as yet to evaluate this exercise, we have much circumstantial evidence showing the benefits for both mother and child. We have found that mothers who consistently practiced this exercise before birth had many more instances of babies presenting head first (vertex position) and in the anterior position (head facing toward the mother's back); significantly diminished incidences of wrapped umbilical cords; and greater ease and satisfaction in the birth process. Babies are born looking calm and alert. Bonding gets off to a better start. Also, the immune systems of both mother and child appear to be enhanced, but we will have to wait for clinical trials to be able to determine that with certainty.

You will also want to practice the correct breathing for labor. Creation starts with a B; that is what the Bible tells us. Its first word "In the beginning" is *Bereshit* in the original Hebrew. The Hebrew B is a curve ending with a line and is called *bet,* which means house. It has a containing space and an opening, as all houses do and as your body does.

Practice saying "beuu" and you will experience how your body curves in at the abdomen, your pelvis rolls forward, and you can easily push, as you would when pushing out a stool. In fact, you can't pronounce the B without breathing out. If you sing it out from deeper and deeper inside you, you will feel your anus and vagina opening up. It is the best sound to sing aloud when you are pushing.

In the first phase of labor return to *Natural breathing* (page 41). Without changing your breathing, concentrate more on your outbreath. Hear it as a smooth *beuu* wind coming out of you. The *beuu* sound is nearly silent.

When we feel pain, we tend to hold our breath. This goes against the truth of your body that is trying to open up. So go with the movement of the body that wants to open up. When the contraction comes, breathe out. Your pain will be greatly reduced.

BEUU BREATHING
exercise 63

Breathe out slowly as if through a long straw that starts way down in your lower abdomen.

Breathe out on the sound of "beuu" very quietly. At first you make this sound in your mouth, then slowly bring it down into your throat, then abdomen. Eventually it should sound like the wind rustling through the leaves of a tree. Try to make the sound very smooth; imagine it as a long, smooth ribbon of dough. Practice this breathing until it feels effortless.

Another way to stay softened and relaxed is with a well-lubricated body that will help you open up and push your baby out more easily. If you are constipated, which is a common complaint in pregnant women, the following exercise will help. Or you can try it on your child, if you have one, when she is having the same difficulty. Do this not only to help your child, but to verify the effectiveness of imagery. It will give you the incentive to continue practicing.

DROP OF OIL
exercise 64

Close your eyes. Breathe out slowly three times, counting from 3 to 1, seeing the numbers in your mind's eye. See the number 1 as tall, clear, and bright.

Imagine catching a ray of sunlight in a small crystal vial. Hold the vial for a moment in your hands. See the sunlight in the vial becoming liquid golden oil.

Breathe out. Drink the oil, seeing it going down into your hips and your pelvic bone structure. See it coating your whole bone structure, then moving into your muscular structure.

Breathe out. See how the sunlit oil begins to expand into all of your pelvic area. See the muscles becoming soft and pliant, the bone structure opening up and breathing with the sunlit oil. See the pelvic floor softening and opening up.

Breathe out. See the drop of oil flowing down into your womb and continuing to expand and soften your tissues. See your cervix opening easily. See the skin of your perineum—supple, golden, and elastic—stretching easily.

Breathe out. Imagine your baby rotating into the right position and, coated in oil, slipping out easily.

Breathe out. Open your eyes.

For passing a stool: See the sunlit oil flow down through your digestive tract to the end of the tube, coating the passage and anal opening with warmth.

The best way to relax into a contraction and breathe naturally is to have someone coach you through your imagery during the contractions. Many women respond best to *Become the water* (page 132) or *Elongate with the movement of the waves* (page 178). Start practicing these exercises now so that you become familiar with and attuned to the images and sensations that need to be elicited when the time comes.

YOUR BIRTH PLAN

It is time to begin really focusing on the kind of birth you have envisioned for yourself. Visualizing the type of birth you want creates the intent. Remember that inception comes before manifestation. What you visualize is what you put into motion. It will be easier to communicate what you want to your doctor, midwife, or doula if you have a clear picture in mind. Seeing it clearly makes it easier to speak about it clearly.

You and your child call the shots here. You are in control. At any time, you can change your plan to suit your needs and those of your child. So when we speak of a birth plan, we know that it is subject to change.

You probably have guessed that I lean toward a natural birth. I believe that your body knows how to give birth. Clearing the way for it to do its job has been my aim throughout these chapters. But what is a natural birth? *It is what is natural for you, and what is natural for your child.* After all, she comes into this world with her own baggage, which is what Buddhists call karma. And so she, too, has a say in how her birth unfolds.

However you define natural birth, you need to let your practitioner know what your preferences are. Here is your checklist:

- Hospital, birthing center, or home birth; water birth
- Doctor or midwife
- Doula or just your partner or coach
- Caesarean or vaginal birth (natural birth)
- Epidural or no pain medication
- Continuous fetal monitoring, intermittent fetal monitoring, or Doppler
- Choosing episiotomy: yes or no
- Postponing cutting the umbilical cord
- Keeping baby with you at all times (not in the common nursery)
- Don't forget to decide what kind of atmosphere you want: for instance dim lights, music, pillows

Do not let this list overwhelm you. If you do the exercises, you will be well prepared to listen to your body and make those decisions. The exercises that follow will help you visualize the different eventualities and choose what seems right and natural for you.

129

Hospital, Birthing Center, or Home Birth; Water Birth

You may not have a choice between hospital, birthing center, or home birth. If you have a high-risk pregnancy, you will have to go to the hospital. High risk doesn't necessarily mean that you or your baby are unhealthy. If you are over thirty-five years old, your practitioner may feel it is safer for you and your baby to be at a medical facility. Some hospitals have a birthing center, which makes both options available to you. You give birth in the birthing center, but if you need medical intervention, the hospital is right there. With a home birth, make sure your midwife has hospital and OB/GYN backup and emergency transport.

If there are no immediate or obvious concerns about safety, the decision will rest with you. What do you want? How do you see your baby's birth? What is more comfortable for you? Visiting the various facilities, asking your friends about their experiences, and reading up on different options are all important. You will, of course, want to discuss your possible choices with your partner, but the choice is ultimately yours to make. The truth of what is most natural and most comfortable for you lies, as always, within you.

DECISION MAKING
exercise 65

Close your eyes. Breathe out slowly three times, counting from 3 to 1, seeing the numbers in your mind's eye. See the number 1 as tall, clear, and bright.

Ask yourself what is the most comfortable and safest way for you to give birth. See what images appear. Accept them, knowing your inside truth has spoken.

Breathe out. Open your eyes.

If you are conflicted, either because of your own issues or because your partner and you do not agree, you may not be able to see and hear what your inside wants. You can always ask your dreams (page 10). Or you may want a stronger exercise.

THE FEATHER OF TRUTH
exercise 66

Close your eyes. Breathe out slowly three times, counting from 3 to 1, seeing the numbers in your mind's eye. See the number 1 as tall, clear, and bright.

Look at Lady Justice. She holds golden scales in her left hand. See her placing the red feather of truth in one scale.

Breathe out. See yourself placing your question—see it as a dream object—in the other scale. If the scale dips, you know the answer is no. If the scales balance, the answer is yes.

Breathe out. Do not try to change or influence what you see. Accept and trust the answer that comes to you from inside yourself.

Breathe out. Open your eyes.

Unless your circumstances change—a new health problem or a complication for you or your child—do not repeat this exercise.

If you choose home birth or a birthing center, you have the option of a water birth. Water births were first popularized by Dr. Michel Odent, a French obstetrician. He had noticed that laboring women seemed to gravitate toward water—their bath or a birthing pool—wherever they could find it. Once in the water, these women didn't want to come out, so he began delivering babies in the water.

Warm water has an analgesic effect on the woman that is "associated with lower levels of stress hormones and increased release of oxytocin," according to Dr. Odent. The research shows that it is as safe to deliver in water as it is to have a regular birth. The water temperature must be maintained at body temperature. Do not enter the pool until you are at least five centimeters dilated; your practitioner will let you know.

As I mentioned, water holds great attraction for women in labor. It helps relax the body and reminds you that letting go and going with the flow will make everything much easier for you. If you are planning on having a water birth, here is the exercise to practice. If you are not, there is even more reason to practice this exercise. It is a wonderful way to prepare yourself for labor.

BECOME THE WATER
exercise 67

Close your eyes. Breathe out slowly three times, counting from 3 to 1, seeing the numbers in your mind's eye. See the number 1 as tall, clear, and bright.

See yourself walking in the countryside, listening to the sounds of water. You come to a brook. It is clear and fresh. Take your clothes off and get into the slow-moving water.

Breathe out. Float, letting the water carry you. At some point, become the water.

Breathe out. As the water begins to move a little faster, relax completely. You are the water. As you slide easily around rocks and obstacles, feel how easy it is to just let go.

Breathe out. Feel yourself flowing into the ocean. Become the ocean.

Breathe out. Feel how easily your baby slips out of you into the ocean.

Breathe out. Become yourself again. Step out of the ocean, holding your baby in your arms.

Breathe out. Look at your baby, smile at her, and see her eyes responding as she smiles back.

Breathe out. Open your eyes, seeing the birth with open eyes.

Doctor or Midwife

Since you had to choose your practitioner early on in your pregnancy, you probably have already decided whether to go with a doctor or midwife. But if you aren't comfortable with your choice, remember that you are always free to change your mind. With a doctor (OB/GYN), you will be giving birth in a hospital; with a midwife, in a birthing center or at home. If you decide on a home birth, make sure the midwife has a working relationship with a team of obstetricians and can gain immediate admission to a hospital near where you live. Hospital backup and emergency transport are an indispensable component of a home birth. This is what makes the Dutch system so impressive. Thirty percent of births there are home births attended by midwives. If the woman requires hospitalization, transport has been arranged in advance at a hospital close by. The midwife attends her there also. Midwives attend 46 percent of Dutch women with low-risk pregnancies. Obstetricians attend the high-risk pregnancies. The system is completely integrated, with midwives and doctors working together, something we don't have in the US. Midwives here are frowned upon, and so are the women who choose home births. So keep that in mind when you make your decision. Then do the *Decision-making* exercise (page 130). If you don't reach a final decision, ask your dreams or do *The feather of truth* exercise (page 131) to determine who your practitioner should be, knowing that your selection will also determine where you give birth.

Doula or Just Your Partner or Coach

Your decision whether to have a doula or just your partner or friend in attendance is important, as your coach will make sure you have the continuous support you need that your doctor or midwife may not have time to provide. You can have both doula and partner, of course. It all depends on your partner's ability to be there for you and to know what to do. I recommend that if you are practicing the imagery, you get a doula trained in DreamBirth to follow you throughout your pregnancy. By the time of your delivery, your body will be highly attuned to the imagery. You will know how to enter into the dream flow effortlessly, and your body will know that your mind is not opposing its efforts to deliver safely. Again and again, women have reported how beneficial the imagery was for them. The advantage of DreamBirth is that you can do the imagery on the phone if there isn't a DreamBirth doula in your area. Many women who practice DreamBirth with their doulas on the phone but don't have them there during labor or delivery go on to have very satisfying birth experiences. Being fully concentrated in their dreaming and assisted by their partner/coach (most often also trained in DreamBirth: see chapter 8, Fathers and Partners) proves to be sufficient.

Here again, you will want to turn inward and ask yourself whether you will be comfortable with only your partner/coach or whether you will need more support. It's all up to you. Do the *Decision making* exercise (page 130) again and ask your dreams or do *The feather of truth* exercise (page 131) to make a final decision about who should be your support and protection in the delivery room.

Caesarean Section Versus Vaginal Birth

This is probably not on your most-popular-subject list, and you would rather not think about it happening to you. Your mind is made up that you will have a vaginal birth. But it is better to be prepared than sorry. If you know how to deal with a Caesarean, it won't be such a shock if your body or your child should require that you have one.

Electing to have a Caesarean—maternal-request Caesareans represent an estimated 2.5 percent of all US births—may make sense to some women, especially if rape or molestation is involved or if her mental or family history make it emotionally difficult for her to deal with childbirth. But she will have to convince her doctor, as the American College of Obstetricians and Gynecologists (ACOG) guidelines support vaginal births unless medically counter-indicated. Other women, however, may have no choice.

A Caesarean is considered both major surgery and a safe procedure. It is still surgery, however, and there are always some risks involved. It also means that you will have to deal with the aftereffects of anesthesia and the wound. In some countries, the rate of Caesareans is very high, notably in Brazil, where the rate in government hospitals is 37 percent, and in private hospitals a shocking 80 percent. In the United States, the latest published rate for Caesareans, while varying from hospital to hospital, is about 34 percent and rising due to a number of factors, some health related and some not. Holland, with a low Caesarean rate of 13.5 percent—and a low infant mortality rate as well (it's among the ten countries with the lowest mortality rate)—shows that the high number of Caesareans in other countries is avoidable.

You will have no choice but to have a Caesarean if you have had previous Caesarean with vertical uterine incision; maternal diabetes or other illnesses; an active herpes infection (if not active, you can give birth vaginally); placenta previa (when the placenta covers the cervical opening); abruptio placenta (when there is separation of the placenta from the uterine wall); preeclampsia (pregnancy induced hypertension); or the size of the baby's head is disproportionate to your pelvis; the fetus presents in breech, foot, or transverse position; or is two or more weeks overdue, and the uterine environment is beginning to deteriorate. When Caesareans for these reasons are preplanned, choose a date that is consistent with family dates (see page 47).

If you are in active labor and your body or the child signals the need for a Caesarean, do not be disappointed. Do not feel that you're a failure. The only failure is a damaged child or mother from not having had a Caesarean when it was medically advisable. Keep in mind that your child's safety is your primary concern. Be glad that there are surgical means of assuring her safety. Remember that you are prepared for just such an eventuality because you have practiced the exercise for Caesareans.

Here are the most frequent reasons for an emergency C-section: failure of labor or of the pushing phase to progress; fetal distress (see exercise *Relief for fetal distress* (page 143); previously undiagnosed problems, such as placenta previa or abruptio placenta; and a prolapsed umbilical cord that, if compressed, could cut off oxygen to the fetus.

Why would you choose to have an elective Caesarean, which is done for nonmedical reasons? Why not a vaginal birth? Fear of the pain of labor: maybe your sister had a very lengthy and painful labor that you witnessed. Fear of the birth process itself: maybe you have a family history that resulted in the near death or death of your mother and grandmother. Esthetics: maybe you're afraid of losing your figure, of becoming flabby. Disgust at the physical process: maybe you have deep ancestral fears or fears arising from your past. One mother who had been raped in her past refused to let her baby be born vaginally, although she was fully dilated and the baby was presenting correctly; she said, "It's dirty down there!" (Try *Emptying your handbag,* page 20, or *Clearing your womb,* page 21, if you have had a similar trauma.)

Doctors will sometimes argue for Caesareans, telling their patients that C-sections are safer than vaginal births. Are they? Not really. It is always best to let nature do what it is meant to do. Many studies have shown that babies delivered naturally have a decided advantage over babies delivered by Caesarean. Due perhaps to the high hormonal exchanges and powerful uterine contractions that help push them through the birth canal, babies born vaginally have stronger immune systems than Caesarean babies, who are likely to develop food sensitivities, diarrhea in the first year, and a greater incidence of slow development. Of course, in the majority of cases, babies delivered by C-sections do perfectly well.

You have already practiced some form of this exercise (*Secret garden,* page 95; you will find the birth version of this exercise, *Drop your weapons,* on page 167). The only two things you must add—and they are of the utmost importance—are asking permission from your body to go ahead with the procedure, and seeing the procedure done perfectly in light.

CAESAREAN
exercise 68

Close your eyes. Breathe out slowly three times, counting from 3 to 1, seeing the numbers in your mind's eye. See the number 1 as tall, clear, and bright.

You are walking around the base of a circular wall. Above the wall, you see the tops of trees. Walk until you find the gate. The key is in the lock: open the gate and walk into the garden.

Breathe out. What does your garden look like? If you're not satisfied with the way it looks, repair your garden.

Breathe out. Walk deeper into the garden and find a patch of very thick, soft, emerald-green grass next to a tree and a running brook.

Breathe out. Lie on the grass in the shade of the tree and listen to the sounds of the brook and the birds. Feel how your body rhythms become attuned to the rhythms of nature.

Breathe out. Now invite those you trust to come into the garden, one by one, and sit in a semicircle around your head. Feel their love and attentiveness.

Breathe out. When all of your witnesses have come in and sat down around you, and when you feel comfortable and at ease, show your body in a precise visualization exactly what is going to happen during the C-section. Ask your body's permission to allow this procedure and remind your body that the C-section is being recommended by your doctor.

Breathe out. If your body refuses permission, ask your body what it needs to make this possible. Respond to the necessity of your body in images.

Breathe out. Once your body has given permission, invite your doctor, assistants, and nurses to come into the garden with their medications and tools. When they stand before you, see how the sunlight pours down onto their heads and into their arms and hands so that everything they touch—medication, tools, your body—turns into light.

Breathe out. See that all is done perfectly. Your baby comes out healthy and whole and is placed on your chest. Smile at your baby and feel that all is well.

Breathe out. When the cord is cut, the placenta lifted away, and your cut stitched up, and the doctor has finished all that must be done, see the doctor, assistants, and nurses leaving.

Breathe out. Feel all of your loved ones still around you, guarding and protecting you; feel their presence and their joy. When you are ready, let them go one by one out of the garden. The gate closes on the last one, and you are alone with your baby and your partner.

Breathe out. Feel the rhythms of nature, feel your body and your baby breathing with the rhythms of nature.

Breathe out. When you are ready, get up with your baby in your arms and, together with your partner, slowly walk out of your garden, close the gate, and take the key or put it in a place where you will always be able to find it.

Breathe out. Walk into your future with your baby in your arms, your partner by your side.

If you know you are going to have a C-section, practice this exercise for three days, three times a day, and on the morning of the procedure.

If you don't plan to have a C-section but want to know what you would do if it were necessary, read this once and ask your partner, doula, or midwife to read it also. They will remember the exercise and be able to take you through it if the doctor decides when you're in labor that you need an emergency C-section. It takes a minute.

Two other exercises should also be done at this time (see appendix 1, page 285). The first, *The river runs through,* is to get rid of the effects of anesthesia and must be done as soon as possible after the procedure, even in the recovery room. The second, *Wound repair 2,* is to help your wound heal faster. Remember these exercises or ask your coach or doula to remember them for you.

Epidural or No Pain Medication

No one wants to suffer pain. Yet the Bible says to the woman, "I will greatly multiply your pain in childbirth. In pain will you bring forth your children."[20] Does this mean we should suffer for the sins of Eve? The overwhelming consensus today is no. We have options.

Today doctors have learned to administer the smallest possible doses for pain relief. The risks are small for both mother and child. The side effects for the mother are that her labor can be slowed down; for the child, that she may be born sluggish and, in rare cases, have difficulty breathing or sucking.

So why not sign up ahead of time for your epidural? The reason is that you may not need one. An epidural is a local anesthetic drug injected in the epidural space to block childbirth pains. You will have no sensations in your pelvis and legs. You will be removed from what is actually happening to you and to your child. With an epidural, you lose control of your body. So why not wait and see? Nobody will refuse you pain medication if you need it or even if you merely want it. So you have time to decide. You can tell your practitioner that you would like an epidural to be available to you if you require it.

Is there a way to deal with pain? Is there a way of mind over body? Exiled in the neocortex, you are acutely "conscious" of the separateness of things, having lost touch with your ability to be at one with your experience. This is what brings about pain.

But you have a way back into your experience: through your dreaming. Dreaming comes from the more ancient and primary structures of the brain, the hypothalamus and pituitary. Dreaming allows you to live fully. Returning to your dreaming means that you are not thinking about your experience but living it. It goes against the grain: who would want to be living their pain? But try "being" your pain and you won't feel it as pain anymore.

"When a woman is in labor, the most active part of her body is her primitive brain . . . There is a reduction in the activity of the brain of the intellect, that is, of the neocortex," says Michel Odent.[21] When you dream or daydream, you are enfolded in your dream, oblivious to your surroundings. You are as uninhibited as you would be at night while living a vivid dream. This is why Dr. Odent advocates that a laboring woman should be left undisturbed unless she requires your presence. If you interrupt her, it is as if you are waking her up from a deep sleep, which can be very disturbing to her. She may not find her rhythm again.

When your rational mind is safely tucked away so that only your dreaming mind is fully engaged and at one with your body, the notion of pain disappears. *What you are experiencing is total presence.* If someone interrupts or frightens you, taking you out of your experience, your level of discomfort is likely to increase. The following exercise sets the intent for your body to disregard such interruptions.

LABOR INTENT
exercise 69

Close your eyes. Breathe out slowly three times, counting from 3 to 1, seeing the numbers in your mind's eye. See the number 1 as tall, clear, and bright.

See a tree made of light, upside down in the sky, its roots floating in the waters of the sky, its trunks and branches of light growing down into your body. See its branches spreading through your lower body, around the uterus, cervix, and perineum.

Breathe out. Tie pink ribbons firmly on each branch so that no message of pain will rise up the tree.

Breathe out. Set a timer to mark your intent. For example, set the timer for forty-eight hours hence.

Breathe out. Decide that when the forty-eight hours are over, the ribbons will dissolve naturally.

Breathe out. Open your eyes.

Setting the time is very important; the subconscious body will obey you. The best way to check on this is to try it with another pain you know you will be experiencing. I did all my dental work that way. For many years, I accepted no anesthetics.

The second exercise is a variant on the *Drop of oil* that Claudia Raiken, one of the doulas in the original group I worked with, uses to deal with pain.

DROP OF OIL FOR
RELEASING CONTRACTIONS
exercise 70

Close your eyes. Breathe out slowly three times, counting from 3 to 1, seeing the numbers in your mind's eye. See the number 1 as tall, clear, and bright.

See your spine and its nerve endings like a beautiful upside-down tree. See the many flowing, graceful branches that supply your pelvic area.

Breathe out. Catch a ray of sunlight in a small crystal vial containing oils. Hold it for a moment, then drink it.

Breathe out. See the oil going down into your hips and pelvic bone structure. Watch as the sunlit oil surrounds, envelops, and coats all the nerve endings in the center of your body, in the pelvic region, and around your womb and cervix. See the oil coat every nerve ending and block all the pain receptors so that all you can feel with each contraction is broad, diffuse pressure.

Breathe out. As surely as oil coats and water flows, only the pressure is sensed and felt—broadly, expansively, easily—until your child is born.

Breathe out. Open your eyes.

Continuous Fetal Monitoring, Intermittent Fetal Monitoring, or Doppler

Fetal monitoring is used to detect your baby's heartbeats and the intensity and duration of your contractions during labor. A strap is wrapped around your abdomen and connected to a monitor. While you are connected to the machine, you are restrained in how you can move. Walking around or getting on your hands and knees is more difficult. You are not uninhibited, free of all restraints, as you should be.

The Doppler is a handheld ultrasound device that amplifies your baby's heartbeats. It replaces the old-fashioned stethoscope that allowed the physician to listen to sounds produced within the body.

The reason your baby's heartbeats need to be monitored is that she is undergoing a strenuous ordeal as she passes through the narrow confines of your pelvic bones. At each contraction, she is being pushed, compressed, constricted. She must wiggle her way through. Fetal distress can occur if she is having trouble with the umbilical cord or placenta or with prolonged labor.

For most low-risk pregnancies, intermittent fetal monitoring is considered sufficient as long as it is used at regular intervals of twenty to thirty minutes during labor. The rest of the time you can move about freely. The Doppler is only used in home births or a birthing center birth.

If there is fetal distress, remember that you can do exercises to communicate with your baby. If you use your images with precision, you can bring about immediate and effective changes in the situation. You have done this basic exercise so many times (*Going into the womb to visit your child,* page 66) that by now it should come naturally to you. Here is a version of it adjusted to just this circumstance.

RELIEF FOR FETAL DISTRESS
exercise 71

Close your eyes. Breathe out slowly three times, counting from 3 to 1, seeing the numbers in your mind's eye. See the number 1 as tall, clear, and bright.

Turn your eyes inward to travel down to your womb. Your eyes shine like two beams illuminating your way. When you are there, look at what is happening to your baby to cause her fetal distress. Address her needs.

Breathe out. Speak to her reassuringly, telling her she is doing fine and that you are there with her.

Breathe out. Reassure her by showing her the way through the birth canal. Keep communicating with her.

Breathe out. Open your eyes.

You have the short version here simply to remind you that you can speak to your baby all through labor and delivery. While your body is working to free her, she is also working to get free and start her journey into this "brave new world."

Choosing Episiotomy: Yes or No

An episiotomy is a small surgical incision made in the perineum from the posterior end of the vulva toward the anus to enlarge the opening for delivery. The cut can be either a midline (vertical) or mediolateral (at an angle) incision. Doctors would perform it to avoid an irregular tear in the mother's perineum that they believed made stitching and healing more difficult. Episiotomies used to be routine in the United States (the American College of Obstetricians and Gynecologists—ACOG—does not support routine use of episiotomies) and are still widely performed in many parts of the world. They were thought to help with the emergence of the baby's head while reducing birth trauma to her skull. Studies have shown that both babies and mothers do better without routine episiotomies and that a natural tear heals better and faster than an episiotomy.

Of course, there are reasons why an episiotomy may need to be performed: if the baby's head is too large; if her shoulder gets stuck in the birth canal (shoulder dystocia); if Pitocin is used to induce labor, which, because contractions come on much faster, increases a woman's chances of serious tearing.

If an episiotomy is required, you will be given a local anesthetic and the incision will not hurt. You won't even know it is being done. Nor will you feel it when being sutured after your baby's birth.

In the US 31 percent of women still receive episiotomies. Keloids (excess growth of scar tissue) can occur after episiotomies, which may result in painful sexual intercourse later on. Tell your doctor or midwife that you prefer not to have an episiotomy if at all possible. Then launch your own preventive program.

Start with asking your partner to help by giving you a perineal massage, using vitamin E oil, around the 34th week. Or you can do it yourself. Once or twice a day for a minute or so should be sufficient. To enhance your physical massage, also do an imaginal massage to soften and stretch your skin.

EGYPTIAN HANDS
exercise 72

Close your eyes. Breathe out slowly three times, counting from 3 to 1, seeing the numbers in your mind's eye. See the number 1 as tall, clear, and bright.

Imagine that you are standing in a very green meadow. The sky is clear and blue. Look up at the sun. Where is the sun? Watch as the sun moves across the sky until it is just above you. If the sun is behind you, turn to face it.

Lift your arms up toward the sun. Feel them stretching, getting longer and longer until your fingers are close to the sun and are very warm and filled with light.

Breathe out. Look at your hands. See that a little hand grows out of the tip of each finger. Now you have fifty little fingers of light at the tips of your fingers.

Breathe out. Bring your arms down to your body. With your fifty little fingers, start massaging the skin of your perineum. Feel your fifty little fingers moving very fast up and down the length of the perineum. See the blood flow into the skin, where it picks up all the cellular toxins while filling the cells with oxygen.

Breathe out. See the blood flow out of the perineum, carrying away the toxins.

Breathe out. See the skin as a stretchy, light material. Stretch it with your fingers of light. Each time you massage, stretch it a little more.

Breathe out. Lift your hands up toward the sun and see your little hands returning into your fingers.

Breathe out. Your hands are full of light. Place them over the perineum. Feel the warmth penetrating your skin, soothing and relaxing that area.

Breathe out. Open your eyes.

Also use the *Drop of oil* exercise (page 127). You can incorporate the two exercises by seeing your hands of light filled with the oil of the sun. Combining these exercises will help enhance the pliability of your skin.

Postponing Cutting the Umbilical Cord

In the Western medical world, the general practice is to clamp and cut the cord immediately after birth. Why would you ask your doctor or midwife to do it differently? Clinical studies have shown that a wait of three minutes allows for the transfer of about 100 mL (3.4 ounces) of blood from the placenta to the newborn, supplying it with extra iron, which may help prevent iron deficiency during the first year after birth.

Ask your doctor or midwife to wait until the cord has finished pulsating strongly (maximum five minutes). Your partner may want to cut the cord. Cutting the cord is a very sacred moment, as it initiates your child's first moment as an entity independent of your body. You may want to mark the moment with a prayer or a ritual.

The cord is attached to the placenta, which you will deliver soon after your child is born. You can ask for the placenta and cord to be saved so you can plant them in a place that feels sacred to you. You may want to have the placenta ground and saved in pill form; it contains many valuable nutrients for you and for your child. If you wish to save the cord and placenta, be sure to tell your birth practitioner ahead of time.

IS BABY IN THE RIGHT POSITION?

Your baby may play havoc with your labor plans if she is not in the optimal head-down position (called vertex) for a safe vaginal delivery. If she is breech (buttocks first, legs flat against the face), footing (one or both legs pointing down), or transverse (lying horizontally, also called shoulder presentation), your obstetrician or midwife will try a hands-on manipulation through your belly, to turn your baby in the desired position. Acupuncture, the age-old Chinese system of using needles and moksa (heat) to help relax and restore the body to its optimal well-being, can also help.

But why not first try changing the baby's position with imagery? Then, if you're successful, you will have verified once again that imagery does work, which should give you a lot of confidence in the language of images you've been learning. You can repeat this exercise if your baby doesn't turn on your first try.

TURNING BABY
exercise 73

Close your eyes. Breathe out slowly three times, counting from 3 to 1, seeing the numbers in your mind's eye. See the number 1 as tall, clear, and bright.

See yourself in a meadow. It's a bright, sunny day.

Breathe out. Stretch your arms out toward the sun, feel them elongating until your hands are very close to the sun. See your hands becoming very warm and turning into light.

Breathe out. Now feel your arms returning to their natural length.

Breathe out. Bring your hands inside your body to the amniotic sac. Gently and carefully take hold of the sac and move it until your baby is in the ideal position for birth: head down and facing toward your back, cord floating up loosely.

Breathe out. Take your hands out of your body and place them on your belly. Send warmth and reassurance to your baby that this is the correct and ideal position for birth.

Breathe out. With open eyes, see your baby in the ideal position for birth.

TRUSTING THE PROCESS OF YOUR BIRTH STORY

You are now ready for the big day. Enjoy this time, as you can now rest and relax, especially if you've stopped working in anticipation of your delivery. All major decisions and purchases have been made; the baby's room is ready.

You can enjoy the satisfaction of knowing you have done every-thing to be consciously prepared for your baby's birth. At night, you will want to relax completely, trusting in your body's ability to regen-erate and prepare for the birth of your child. Here is a simple "visual prayer" to use if you believe in a higher power. Practice it at night before going to sleep.

IN THE HAND OF THE DIVINE
exercise 74

Close your eyes. Breathe out slowly three times, counting from 3 to 1, seeing the numbers in your mind's eye. See the number 1 as tall, clear, and bright.

See a divine hand coming down from heaven. Step into the hand and lie back. Feel that both you and your child are supported and protected.

Breathe out. Continue seeing this as you fall asleep.

If you are not a believer, you can replace *In the hand of the Divine* with the *Ocean of light* exercise.

OCEAN OF LIGHT (2)
exercise 75

Close your eyes. Breathe out slowly three times, counting from 3 to 1, seeing the numbers in your mind's eye. See the number 1 as tall, clear, and bright.

See before you an ocean of golden light. Step into it and lie back, floating on the ocean of golden light. Feel that both you and your child are supported and protected.

Breathe out. Continue seeing this as you fall asleep.

Read the next two chapters on labor and bonding now, as you will be too busy when labor is upon you and when baby has arrived. You have practiced most of the exercises for labor ahead of time. The bonding exercises (chapter 7) may be of help right now to assuage your fears about motherhood if you have any. Seeing ahead is a good practice and always makes things easier because you already know the way.

You have now done all that you can do to fully prepare for the great day. Your mind is educated as to your options; your emotions have been examined and transformed to the best of your ability; and your body is informed and practiced, through the visual exercises, to perform at its peak. After your baby is born, time will be in short supply. If you are first-time parents, make sure to cherish these last days of freedom. Congratulate yourself on a journey well traveled, and take the time to savor moments of peace and togetherness with your partner before Baby arrives.

PART THREE

❦

Welcoming Your Baby

6

The Flower Opens

Whoever is soft and yielding
Is a disciple of life.

TAO TSE CHING

YOU ARE APPROACHING the last leg of the race. Like Demeter—
meter, mother, mistress, wise one of abundance—you are readying
your *de,* doorway, for the advent of your child. You are both subject
and initiator: stretching open that doorway to let your child through,
like the Creatrix, to expel the creation that you housed and nurtured
for nine long months. The initiator is not your conscious mind, the
mind that thinks it knows and has been told by the doctor what your
due date is. It is your body supreme, that magnificent subconscious
intelligence that, in concert with your child's elemental intelligence,
has determined the release of the trigger. The beginnings may be slow,
a few days or weeks. The momentum builds up and gathers energy. It
will intensify and reach a climax. You will know then that the birth
of your baby is imminent. All of your pent-up emotions, your nine
months of preparation, your hopes and expectations, become laser-
focused on accomplishing the task at hand—delivering your baby.

To bring forth is a miraculous occurrence. Enjoy it. You have no
choice. You're on a roller coaster. If you tense up, the thrill of going

153

over the top, plunging down, and rising up again will be drowned by your fear. Staying with your sensations—remaining, as it were, on top of them—will allow you to be fully present during the ride. If you hold back, you are opposing a will far stronger than yours. This is the life force taking over, and like all elemental forces, it will thunder and roll through you. Surrender, let go, and go with the flow. At some point toward the end, when you are completely subsumed and at one with this elemental force, you will use it to push your child out. It will give you a tremendous sense of your innate power and accomplishment.

At the moment of birth, having lost all inhibitions, all petty fears and concerns, you are completely in the now of your business. You cannot comprehend yet the shock of revelation and joy that awaits you. Soon you will gaze upon the face of your child. He will open eyes of unfathomable depth and purity. You will fall into his mystery, tumbling into love, and be filled with heart-stopping joy, like Sarah who gave birth to her son and called him *Laughter* (Itzhak).

LIGHTENING AND ENGAGEMENT

Two to four weeks before you give birth to a first baby, or closer to labor if this is not your first pregnancy, your baby drops down into your pelvic cavity. This is called lightening—probably because having more room to breathe and digest, you feel lighter. Conversely, you will feel an increased pressure on your pelvic floor and bladder, which means you will have to pee more often. The baby drops when the cervix starts to thin, a sure sign that you are approaching your final weeks. At the same time, you'll be experiencing more vaginal secretions. If your discharge is pinkish and glutinous, you know that your mucous plug, which closed your cervix during pregnancy, has come loose. It is one of the signs of approaching labor.

When your baby starts descending through the pelvic bones, it will be apparent just by looking at your lowered baby bump. Your partner and your friends will be able to observe it. You'll know because your sense of balance shifts. This is as it should be.

But what if your baby isn't dropping? Can you do something about it? Are you overdue? Some women have longer pregnancies, especially if it is a first baby. Being overdue as much as two weeks is not out of the ordinary. After the 42nd week, your doctor may find it medically necessary to induce labor. Why not try to do something about it, as a baby who doesn't engage means you may be heading for a C-section? To get your baby to drop, gravity is your first tool: walk. But also use what should by now be a trusted and familiar tool: your imagery. Remembering your main exercise of the last three months, *Rehearsing the birth—the flower* (page 124), practice seeing your baby entering the stem of the upside-down flower.

LIGHTENING
exercise 76

Close your eyes. Breathe out slowly three times, counting from 3 to 1, seeing the numbers in your mind's eye. See the number 1 as tall, clear, and bright.

See your baby—head down, facing back, cord floating freely—beginning to descend through the open stem of the birthing flower.

Breathe out any fear or anxiety as a dark smoke. See the smoke becoming lighter and lighter. On the inhale, see yourself breathing the golden light of the sun. See it like golden oil coating your baby's skin, then pouring down the inside of the stem.

Breathe out. See your baby slipping easily down the funnel of the stem and slowly sliding farther and farther down until his head touches the opening of the flower.

Breathe out, knowing that the flower has its own rhythm and will open up slowly but surely to let your baby through.

Breathe out. Open your eyes.

I taught this exercise to a woman who had to be induced three weeks before her due date because of meconium staining (observed when amniotic fluids are colored, which indicates that your baby has had a bowel movement, a sign that he may be in distress). The doctor was sure the baby wouldn't drop, which meant she'd have to have a C-section. We also did the exercise for her, visualizing her baby dropping. In one hour, the baby had engaged completely—to the doctor's amazement—and her labor progressed normally. She gave birth vaginally to a wonderful baby boy.

FALSE LABOR AND WHAT TO DO WHILE YOU WAIT

If you feel a tightening of the uterus at irregular intervals—generally painless—you are experiencing practice contractions, called Braxton Hicks contractions or false labor. You will know for sure that this is not true labor if changing your position stops the contractions.

Is there such a thing as false labor? Not really. These contractions are called false labor because they are not strong enough to induce labor. But they do begin the process of effacement and dilation of the cervix (thinning out and opening of the cervix). That means your practitioner may tell you at your next visit that you've already begun dilating. You're giving yourself a head start, but you're not in labor yet.

You'll know when you're in labor because your contractions will start coming more frequently and at regular intervals, building in intensity. Before this happens, it might be time to check over your exercises, especially *Rehearsing the birth—the flower* (page 124) (or *Caesarean* on page 137 if you have planned for a C-section), *Blue vase* (page 100), *Drop of oil for releasing contractions* (page 141), and *Become the water* (page 132).

Your body is a marvelous tool that subconsciously takes care of all your needs. It breathes, digests, excretes, perspires, pumps blood, and sends messages without your being involved in a conscious way. Your body knows what it needs. Treating it with respect is like taking care of your favorite pet. If you love it, it responds in a well-behaved way.

If you neglect it, it may bite. Your next exercise is about asking your body what it needs to be fully prepared for the birth experience.

ASKING IF THE BODY IS READY FOR BIRTH
exercise 77

Close your eyes. Breathe out slowly three times, counting from 3 to 1, seeing the numbers in your mind's eye. See the number 1 as tall, clear, and bright.

Turn your eyes inward, seeing the light of your eyes illuminating the inside of your body. Ask each part of your body, one by one, if it is ready for birth. If a part of your body is not ready, ask for an image that shows you what needs to be addressed. Then respond to the needs of that image.

Spine—breathe out
Shoulders—breathe out
Rib cage—breathe out
Pelvis—breathe out
Cervix—breathe out
Uterus—breathe out
Vagina—breathe out
Hips—breathe out
Legs—breathe out
Feet—breathe out
And any other part of your body you feel impelled to ask.

Breathe out. Open your eyes.

Here is an example of an exercise that might address your hips' need for extra attention and tender loving care before labor starts in earnest, as they will need to widen and open to facilitate your baby's passage through the birth canal.

FREE UP THE LOWER BACK AND PELVIS
exercise 78

Close your eyes. Breathe out slowly three times, counting from 3 to 1, seeing the numbers in your mind's eye. See the number 1 as tall, clear, and bright.

Imagine you are in a meadow. Look up at the sky. Where is the sun? If it's to your left, watch it as it moves across the sky until it reaches midheaven.

Breathe out. Stretch your arms up toward the sun. Feel them getting longer and longer. Feel the warmth of the sun turn your hands into light.

Breathe out. Bring your hands of light down into your body. Delicately spread apart the hip bones from the inside.

Breathe out. Take your hands out and place them on your hips, sensing the warmth and light of your hands seeping into your pelvic area.

Breathe out and open your eyes.

WILL THE OPENING BE WIDE ENOUGH?

Your body is made to bring children into the world. You may be one of those women who are too small or whose baby's head is disproportionately large for your pelvic bones (cephalopelvic disproportion). If that's the case, you will already have been advised by your doctor, who will have scheduled a C-section for you. But, as the French say, the exception confirms the rule—which means that you are likely large enough for your baby to pass through. The exercise *Rehearsing the birth—the flower* (page 124), in which you see the flower opening wider and wider, will support your body in doing its job of opening up. You can think of it and the following exercises as reverse Kegel exercises (page 228).

The ancients have another secret hidden in plain sight that will help the cervix open up. In all the ancient sacred languages, the word for doorway starts with a D: Greek, *de;* Hebrew, *dalet;* Sanskrit, *dwr;* Celtic, *duir.* This has carried forward all the way to our own English word, *door.* Doorways have been seen as passageways that are sacred to women and often painted red.

DEMETER, DOORWAY OF THE MYSTERIOUS FEMININE
exercise 79

Breathe out on the sound *de.* Keep the sound high, *deeee . . .* holding the sound as long as is comfortable. If you pay attention, you will feel all your lower parts opening, from the inside out. Feel how your vulva opens up.

Let the breath in. See it as golden light that flows down to your cervix and vulva, coating them with golden warm sunlight.

Repeat three times.

Breathe out. Open your eyes.

This exercise is for opening the cervix, not for pushing. We will review the exercise for pushing with its distinctive, loud *beuuu* sound when the time comes. Practice this exercise during the last three weeks before your due date or until and when labor begins. Do not practice it anytime earlier.

Other exercises for opening include *Duck breath* and *The peach*.

Your body is made in twos, like a mirror image of itself. Your left side is a mirror image of your right side. Your lower half is a mirror image of your top half. That means the openings in your face and the openings in your perineum are intimately connected. If an opening above is tense, the corresponding opening below will also be tense. If your mouth is loose, so will your vulva be loose.

DUCK BREATH
exercise 80

Breathe out through loose lips, blowing out repeatedly, vibrating your lips and letting them flap open. Visualize your lips flapping. Sense and see what is happening in your vulva.

You want to loosen up more than your lips or vulva. Here is another exercise to relax and open up the inside of your mouth. Watch how it also affects the inside of your uterus and cervix.

THE PEACH
exercise 81

Close your eyes. Breathe out slowly three times, mouth slightly open, lips loose, counting from 3 to 1, seeing the numbers. See the 1 as tall, clear, and bright.

Breathe out. You are walking in a peach orchard. Pick a small peach, warm from the sun, and put it whole into your mouth. Feel it growing and growing until it is huge in your mouth.

Breathe out. Sense and see what is happening in the lower regions and openings of your body.

Breathe out. Now the peach is melting in your mouth. Taste its golden juices. Sense and see them flowing down to coat the insides of your uterus and cervix.

Breathe out. Sense the roughness of the peach pit against your tongue. Now, pursing your lips, spit it out.

Breathe out. Open your eyes.

The more you relax, the faster you will open up. As I write this, an email just came in that said, "Our son was born yesterday. The exercises we have done helped us a lot. Everything was very fast . . . opening from 3 cm to 8 cm in one hour!"

TRUE LABOR

If you feel a sudden rush of water between your legs, it means that your water bag (the membrane containing the amniotic fluids in which your baby has floated for nine months) has just ruptured. If so, you can expect your first true contractions in the next twelve to twenty-four hours. Call your practitioner when your water bag breaks. For some women the membrane might not rupture until labor starts. If the bag hasn't broken spontaneously, your doctor will decide whether to rupture it (you won't feel it) or to let your baby be born in the bag. It will then be ruptured so your baby can take his first breath.

Do not be worried about breaking your waters in public. It rarely happens because when you're standing or sitting, your baby's head blocks the passage. It's more likely to happen when you're lying down.

The amniotic fluid is pale and gushes out quite quickly. The sensation is different from an involuntary release of urine. When your waters break, remind yourself to do the water birthing exercise, *Become the water* (page 132).

There are three stages to labor:

Stage one is labor. It has three distinctive phases: 1) early labor, when the cervix thins and dilates to 3 centimeters (early labor can happen in the last three weeks of pregnancy or in just a few short hours); 2) active labor, when the cervix dilates to 7 centimeters; 3) transitional labor, when the cervix dilates to 10 centimeters. It is when you are reaching complete dilation that you may feel overwhelmed and say, "I can't go on!" Have your partner/coach remind you that you are nearly at the pushing stage. In labor, all you have to do is ride the wave of your contractions. Your body and your baby's body are doing all the work.

Stage two is pushing and delivering your baby. Here you do the work in tandem with your contractions. While the uterus works strongly on its own to expel Baby, your pushing facilitates and accelerates the process. A strong, active push on your part during a contraction will be a lot more effective than the contraction alone. And the truth is that both you and Baby need this stage to proceed as quickly as possible.

Stage three is the delivery of the placenta. Contractions are mild, and often you don't even feel its expulsion.

You are officially in labor when your contractions come at regular intervals and build up in intensity. Your partner/coach can time the interval between contractions, starting from the beginning of one contraction and going to the beginning of the next.

During labor, you may find that all of the exercises you were about to do will be wiped out of your mind as your body takes over. Don't worry about it. As long as you practiced the exercises ahead of time, your subconscious will have integrated them, and your body will follow the instructions you have given your subconscious.

Stage One: The Three Phases of Labor

Early Stage of Labor

In the early phase of labor, try to sleep or make yourself comfortable. If you feel restless and want to busy yourself about the house, don't hold back. In fact, you've probably been very busy in the last twenty-four hours, engaged in what is called the "nesting instinct," also a reliable sign that labor is imminent. You will want to attend to all the last details before Baby comes so you can be free to concentrate on giving birth. Resting, relaxing, or busying yourself are all good ways to get yourself through this phase of labor. If you're hungry, eat a light meal and drink to sustain yourself as you burn calories during active labor. And don't forget to urinate frequently.

Resting and relaxing are best done in a quiet place.

QUIET PLACE
exercise 82

Close your eyes. Breathe out slowly three times, mouth slightly open, lips loose, counting from 3 to 1, seeing the numbers. See the 1 as tall, clear, and bright.

Go to a quiet and safe place where you feel at ease, or to your secret garden.

Stay in that place for a moment. Where are you? What does it look like, feel like? Describe it to yourself.

Breathe out. Open your eyes, seeing the place with open eyes.

If you have been very busy applying the last touches to your home, do this exercise once you've finished.

READIED HOME
exercise 83

Close your eyes. Breathe out slowly three times, mouth slightly open, lips loose, counting from 3 to 1, seeing the numbers. See the 1 as tall, clear, and bright.

See your home as clean and orderly. Put the last touches on your home. You may want to move some things around.

Breathe out. When you are satisfied, go out into your meadow and pick a bouquet of wildflowers. Breathe in their fresh scent and enjoy their colors. Place them in a vase in your home.

Breathe out. Step back and enjoy the sight of what you have accomplished.

Breathe out. Open your eyes, seeing the vase of flowers in your readied home with open eyes.

You have cleaned and readied your home. Now you will want to purify yourself in preparation for this sacred and most holy event. The following exercise is based on ancient purification rituals you'll recognize whether you're a Christian, a Jew, a Muslim, or a Hindu. It consists of complete immersion in a pool of running water that cleanses you of all your sins and returns you to innocence.

IMMERSION
exercise 84

Close your eyes. Breathe out slowly three times, counting from 3 to 1, seeing the numbers in your mind's eye. See the number 1 as tall, clear, and bright.

You are standing next to a deep natural pool fed by a natural spring.

Breathe out. Take your clothes off. Put them in a pile by the pool where you can find them.

Breathe out. Step into the water and immerse yourself completely until not a hair on your head touches the surface of the water. Say a prayer to be cleansed of all that still holds you back from giving birth happily and easily. Come back to the surface.

Breathe out. Immerse yourself a second time, going deeper. See and feel the clear cool waters all around you. Say a prayer to surrender to your body's process and go with the flow.

Breathe out. Immerse yourself a third time, going very deep. Listen to the silence. Feel sustained by the waters all around you. Say a prayer to become one with the womb of the Divine Mother so that she may lend you her strength.

Breathe out. Step out of the pool. Stretch yourself in the sunshine, sing, and dance until you are dry.

Breathe out. Your old clothes have disappeared. New clothes are awaiting you, loose and pastel or white. Put them on. How is your hair? Wet or dry, long or short, or the same? What is your expression?

Breathe out. Open your eyes, seeing yourself dressed in your new clothes.

Active Stage of Labor

When your contractions are four minutes apart and regular, or at least intense—every forty to sixty seconds, with a peak intensity in the middle—you have reached the active phase of labor. As contractions come on faster and more intensely, think of each new contraction as a wave you are surfing. Ride the wave. It rises, it peaks, and it falls. You rest in the valley. It rises and peaks and falls again; you rest. Resting can mean lying down, moving your body freely, dancing, or whatever makes you comfortable.

RIDING THE WAVE (1)
exercise 85

As the contraction begins, blow out a light smoke as well as any tension, fear, or pain you may have.

Looking up at the blue-gold dome of the sky. Let this blue-gold light enter your nostrils, then flow down your back and into your womb, filling your womb. Sense and see your abdomen arching up like the dome of the sky.

Breathe out slowly. Breathe in the blue-gold light, and see it traveling down, softening, relaxing, and coating with blue-gold light your cervix, vulva, hips, thighs, and legs.

Return to your natural breathing, enjoying the pause after the surge and knowing that all is in order and very good.

During the rest period, remember to practice lying back on an *Ocean of light* (page 109) or *In the hand of the Divine* (page 149). Or go into your garden. Here is a little something to add to your *Secret garden* exercise (page 95), in case you are tempted to give in to angry, resentful or self-pitying emotions, which can happen to all of us when we experience discomfort. Giving in to these emotions will only take you out of sync with what is happening to your body and make your discomfort harder to bear. But if you return to your dreaming, the emotions and discomfort will dissolve as you concentrate. Athletes call this "being in the zone." They describe it as a heightened state of consciousness in which time stands still and everything they do is effortless and perfect. It is a "special place where performance is exceptional and consistent, automatic and flowing. An athlete is able to ignore all the pressures and let his or her body deliver the performance that has been learned so well."[22]

DROP YOUR WEAPONS
exercise 86

Close your eyes. Breathe out slowly three times, mouth slightly open, lips loose, counting from 3 to 1, seeing the numbers. See the 1 as tall, clear, and bright.

See yourself standing at the gate of your enclosed garden. You know that the only way to get into your garden is to let fall all your weapons. Hear the sound as they drop to the ground. When the last weapon has fallen to the ground, see the gate opening of its own accord.

Breathe out. What does your garden look like?

Breathe out. Walk deeper into the garden and find a patch of very thick, soft, emerald-green grass next to a shade tree and a running brook.

Breathe out. Lie on the grass in the shade and listen to the sounds of the brook and the birds. Feel how your body rhythms become attuned to the rhythms of nature. Feel the green soothing aura of nature surrounding you and your baby.

Breathe out. Now invite the women of your ancestry and the women friends you trust into the garden to sit behind you. Feel their love and attentiveness to you. Feel the Divine Mother's presence supporting you. Lie back in Her arms.

Breathe out. Once again, rehearse your baby's birth, showing him the stem of the flower. Show your baby how he is going to slide easily and perfectly down the stem and out the wide-open flower into the circle of love that awaits him.

Breathe out. Now invite your doctor and nurses or midwife to come into the garden. When they stand before you, see the sunlight pouring down onto their heads and into their arms and hands so that everything they touch—medication, tools, your body—turns into light.

Breathe out. See your baby being born perfectly and easily. See your baby coming out healthy and whole. See your partner catching the baby and placing him on your chest. Feel how all is well with you and your baby.

Breathe out. See the doctor and nurses or midwife leaving.

Breathe out. Feel all of your loved ones still around you, guarding and protecting you; feel their presence and their joy. When you are ready, let them go one by one out of the garden. The gate closes on the last one, and you are alone with your baby and your partner.

Breathe out. Feel the rhythms of nature; feel your body and your baby breathing with the rhythms of nature.

Breathe out. When you are ready, get up and, with your baby in your arms and your partner by your side, slowly walk out of your garden. Hear the gate closing behind you.

Breathe out. Walk into your future with your baby in your arms, your partner by your side.

Remember that you are the heroine of this dream. Do not judge yourself or put yourself down; rather, decide how you want this story to unfold. Drama, hysteria, fear, and discouragement have no place in your scenario. You are the dreamer manifesting the courage to stay attuned and flexible. You have practiced, and you are ready. If you fall out of rhythm, you can always practice dancing.

RHYTHM
exercise 87

Close your eyes and breathe out three times, hearing a waltz being played.

Listen to the three-beat rhythm. Feel yourself dancing the waltz with your partner—your feet, your whole body dancing to the rhythm of the waltz.

Breathe out. Feel your partner's hand on the small of your back, supporting you and guiding you to the rhythm of the music.

Breathe out. Open your eyes, hearing the music with open eyes and feeling your partner's hand on the small of your back.

In between contractions, during your rest period, remember to return to *Natural breathing* (page 41). This will help center you and clear your emotions. If your breathing is off kilter, you may want to ask your partner or doula to put his or her hand on your chest and urge you to stop breathing there and instead to breathe in your belly. If you breathe out slowly until you are empty, the breath comes in of its own accord and will return to its natural rhythm. If you are calm, you will have returned to your natural breathing. Your coach will calm his or her breathing to allow you to use his or hers as a model. Following is a deepening version of *Natural breathing*. You can choose to do only the first part of the exercise or, if that is not sufficient to calm and refocus you, continue the exercise.

DEEPENING NATURAL BREATHING
exercise 88

Close your eyes. Watch your breathing without trying to change it, allowing your breath to return to its natural rhythm . . . knowing that when your breath returns to its natural rhythm, what is not in place tends to return to be in place.

Bring your attention into your body. Watch your breathing again. Allow it to return to its natural rhythm . . . knowing that when your breath returns to its natural rhythm, what is not in place tends to return to be in place.

Bring your attention deeper into your body. Watch your breathing again. Allow it to return to its natural rhythm . . . knowing that when your breath returns to its natural rhythm, what is out of order tends to return to be in order. Continue doing this until you feel very still and relaxed.

Breathe out. Open your eyes.

If your emotions are still playing havoc with your concentration, remember to sweep them off to the left (*Sweep the porch,* page 75).

Going to the Hospital or Birthing Center

You will know that you need to go to the hospital or birthing center when you feel that you can't see straight any longer. Ina May Gaskin, one of the world's most renowned authors on natural-birth midwifery (and a midwife herself), refers to this moment as "psychedelic." Hopefully the way is short and the car comfortable. If you are truly in a trance, try to stay that way, turned in to yourself. If you are anxious about the drive, do this simple visualization.

BLUE PATHWAY
exercise 89

Breathe out all that tires you, obscures you, upsets you as a dark smoke that floats out of the window and is absorbed by the outside vegetation.

Breathe in the blue-gold light of the sky. See it entering your nostrils, filling your throat and your mouth.

Breathe the blue-gold light slowly out of your mouth, creating a path of blue-gold light all the way from your home to the hospital. See the blue-gold light arriving at the hospital and, as the door opens, entering and filling your birthing room.

Breathe out. See yourself in the car following this path of light to the hospital, knowing that it opens the way and guides you safely from home all the way to your destination. See yourself arriving safely and being welcomed into the birthing room, filled with blue-gold light, where you will continue to labor peacefully.

Breathe out. Open your eyes.

If you are planning a home birth, use this exercise to create greater privacy in your own home. Wherever you are, filling the room with light will provide you and those around you with an instant aura of protection and calm.

THE COCOONED ROOM
exercise 90

Close your eyes. Breathe out slowly three times, counting from 3 to 1, seeing the numbers in your mind's eye. See the number 1 as tall, clear, and bright.

Reach your arm out the window and up toward the sun. Catch a ray of light and wrap it around yourself from your feet to your head. See yourself in a cocoon of light.

Breathe out. Reaching for another ray of light, toss it onto the walls of your room, seeing the room turn to light.

Breathe out. See everything you touch turn into light. See the midwife's or doula's hands, tools, and medications turning into light. Know that with this light, you and your baby are safe and protected from all harm.

Breathe out. Open your eyes.

If you are uncomfortable during your transfer to the hospital or at any other time, voice your concern. If you are disturbed by other people's presence, voice, or touch, say so. If some preoccupation or unresolved emotion surfaces, bring it up. Left unresolved, these concerns can have the effect of slowing down your labor. At this time, when you are so open and vulnerable, you need positive, life-affirming people around you. Remember that what you are doing is a labor of love.

Ask for and insist on loving, supportive people around you. Reconnect and anchor yourself in love.

RETURN TO A PLACE OF LOVE
exercise 91

Close your eyes. Breathe out slowly three times, counting from 3 to 1, seeing the numbers in your mind's eye. See the number 1 as tall, clear, and bright.

Take three steps back into a place of peace, comfort, and beauty, such as your bedroom at home.

Watch your breath, allowing it to return to its natural rhythm, knowing that when your breath returns to its natural rhythm, what is not in order tends to return to be in order.

Sense the place of harmony where you feel quiet and happy.

Breathe out. Return to the first time you fell in love. Feel it.

Breathe out. Send the feeling of love as a bridge of light from your heart to your partner's heart. If you need to say something to your partner, say it now, sending it over the bridge of light.

Breathe out. Open your eyes. Voice your love aloud to your partner.

Sending messages "through the airways" is much more effective than talking. In my practice, I have often seen near-instantaneous resolution of conflict using this method. By resolving to step away from the "story" and return to your heart, you restore sanity and joy to relationships with loved ones.

Don't forget to also voice what you have felt. It will transform the atmosphere of the room. Remember that everything surrounding you must be filled with light and love. Don't be afraid to say, "I love you!" or "Thank you!" If you feel like kissing your partner or having him rub your nipples, do so, advises Ina May Gaskin. It helps activate labor. Some women are very turned on during labor. After all, the same love energy that implanted your baby in your womb also helps to birth him.

Try also to laugh, as Sarah laughed giving birth to her son. Remember that you are not alone with your laboring body. You are surrounded by your loved ones and helpers and by invisible beings you are connected to through a web of love and shared experience. All your women friends who are mothers, all your female ancestors know what it is to give birth and can be emotionally present with you. The divine feminine energy sustains you. I call this the birthing dreamfield.

THE BIRTHING DREAMFIELD
exercise 92

Close your eyes. Breathe out slowly three times, counting from 3 to 1, seeing the numbers in your mind's eye. See the number 1 as tall, clear, and bright.

See yourself as the center of a web of light. At each intersection of the web is a sustaining member of your community of friends, mothers, and ancestors.

Breathe out. Hear them chanting their love. Feel the strands of the web vibrating with their chant of love. Feel what this does to your body and to your baby.

Breathe out. Open your eyes, seeing the love with open eyes.

Refresh your memory by reviewing *Ancestry support* (page 112). Remember that all those who love you, even though they cannot be in the room with you, are with you in their thoughts, prayers, and good wishes.

I remember a single mother who came from Rwanda. Her dead mother, her grandmother, and all the sheep and cattle on her grandmother's land were in the room urging, bleating, mooing. The ancestors were beating their drums. Cheered on by her lost community and family, she gave birth to her son, the new coming from the loss of the old, massacred in the Rwanda genocide. It was a triumph of life over the grim terrors and grief of her past.

Transitional Labor

When your cervix is dilated to 8 cm, you have reached the most intense part of your labor. This transition phase is generally short, no longer than fifteen minutes to an hour. The contractions are close together, and peaks are long. This is the phase where you will want to remember or be talked through the *Blue vase* exercise (page 100), modified to help you go with the waves of sensations that come with contractions.

RIDING THE WAVE (2)
exercise 93

As the contraction begins, blow out dark smoke and with it any pain, tension, or fear you have. See the smoke being absorbed by the vegetation outside.

Inhale the golden light from the sky, seeing it flow, warm and comforting, into your body—melting, softening, widening all that it touches.

Sense and see it melting, softening, widening your forehead; melting, softening, widening your jaw; melting, softening, widening your shoulders . . . chest . . . abdomen. See the light spreading out, flowing into your womb, coating your womb with melting, softening, warm golden light. See the warm golden light surrounding your baby's head, melting the cervix, melting the vaginal muscles, the perineum, inner thighs, calves, and feet.

Breathe out and return to your natural breathing, feeling the pause after the surge and knowing that all is well and in order.

Your partner and/or doula can read this exercise aloud. Ask them to lengthen the pronunciation of the words "melting," "softening," "widening." This will help you to ride the waves of sensation that come with each new contraction. Ask them to do this imagery with you or for you, if you're too engaged. Ask them also to support your lower back with their hands. Feel the warmth and love their hands are communicating to you.

Between contractions, remember to catch a pause. Even a few seconds of resting will reenergize you.

WHITE CLOUD
exercise 94

Close your eyes. Breathe out slowly three times, counting from 3 to 1, seeing the numbers in your mind's eye. See the number 1 as tall, clear, and bright.

Imagine being in a large, quiet, clear open space. Look at a beautiful, round, bright white cloud. Time yourself to the rhythm of this bright white cloud.

Breathe out. Put all your fears, anxieties, or pains in the cloud.

Breathe out. Watch the cloud float away to the left. Feel free of any heaviness or emotional difficulty.

Breathe out. Open your eyes.

You may prefer to alternate the preceding exercise, *Riding the wave (2),* with the next exercise or simply use the one that works best for you. Again, have your partner or doula talk you through it. This exercise reminds you that you are 85-percent water and can flow with the rhythm and fluidity of water. Practice it, like all other exercises in this chapter, before your time of labor so that your body is familiar with the language and follows it effortlessly.

❦

ELONGATE WITH THE
MOVEMENT OF THE WAVES
exercise 95

Close your eyes. Breathe out slowly three times, counting from 3 to 1, seeing the numbers in your mind's eye. See the number 1 as tall, clear, and bright.

Sense, see, and feel that you are on a mountain slope. You have stepped into a rushing mountain stream. Sense the coolness of the water, the sudden rush of the current knocking you off your feet.

Breathe out. Instead of resisting, let go and become one with the rushing stream. Don't be afraid of obstacles because now you are the water. Just flow until you begin to feel that you are slowing down, meandering, spreading out as you approach the ocean. Expand out to become the ocean.

Breathe out. Now feel yourself returning to your body, floating on the ocean. Sense how the ocean is supporting you.

Breathe out. Feel the little wavelets of the quiet ocean traveling all the way down your back from your head to your legs, feet, and toes, elongating your arms and fingers, until you sense and see yourself becoming like a great burst or star of light spread out across the surface of the ocean. Feel the sunlight flowing into you, nourishing every cell of your body. Sense, see, and feel being completely open. See your baby easily slipping out of you and swimming around like a little fish in the ocean.

Breathe out. Once again, return to your natural form, retaining some of your elongation and sense of being rested.

Breathe out. Holding your baby in your arms, float back to shore on your back.

Breathe out. When you are dry, catch a ray of sunlight and wrap yourself and your baby in robes of rainbow light.

Breathe out. Open your eyes.

Fetal Distress

If your baby is experiencing fetal distress at any time during labor, bring your eyes down to speak to him, exactly as you've done for the last nine months. This is often all it takes to calm your baby, whose heartbeats will immediately return to normal.

If the doctor or midwife tells you that the umbilical cord is wrapped tightly around him, making it impossible for him to move down or to breathe, do the following exercise immediately. If you already know how to turn your hands into light, skip the first two inductions. Start with "bringing your hands of light into your womb."

LOOSEN THE CORD
exercise 96

Close your eyes. Breathe out slowly three times, counting from 3 to 1, seeing the numbers in your mind's eye. See the number 1 as tall, clear, and bright.

See yourself in a green meadow. It is a bright and sunny day. Stretch your arms up toward the sun, elongating your arms until your hands are very close to the sun. Now they become very warm and turn into light.

Breathe out. Feel your arms returning to their natural length.

Breathe out. Bring your hands of light into your womb. See the warmth and light touching your baby, illuminating your womb. See your fingers of light gently slipping under the cord and loosening it. Move the cord. See it floating freely from your baby to the placenta.

Breathe out. Make eye contact with your baby, smile, and talk to him, telling him all is well now and he can easily slide through the birth canal coated in the oil of the sun.

Breathe out. See him being born perfectly.

Breathe out. Open your eyes.

Soon you will sense a strong urge to push. Wait until you have been given the go-ahead by your practitioner; you shouldn't start pushing until the cervix is fully dilated. It is common at this point to cry out that you can't do this anymore, that you want an epidural, which the doctor cannot give you at this point. Ask your partner or your doula to remind you that feeling overwhelmed is typical of the short transition moment you're in just now. It'll soon be over and you'll be entering the second stage of labor, where your collaboration is essential and you will be pushing with all your might.

Stage Two: Pushing and Delivery

Suddenly the raging storm of furiously paced contractions is over. You will be surprised at the quiet that follows. You now have time to rest because your contractions are interspaced with well-defined pauses. Practice *Ocean of light (2)* (page 149), *In the hand of the Divine* (page 149), or *White cloud* (page 177) to help you rest and recoupe your energy. On the rise of a contraction, you will be encouraged to push. Do not push when you are not having contractions. When pushing, summon all your fearlessness and courage and give it all you have. Shame and inhibitions have no place in the birthing room and should be discarded like old clothes.

DISCARDING
exercise 97

Close your eyes. Breathe out slowly three times, counting from 3 to 1, seeing the numbers in your mind's eye. See the number 1 as tall, clear, and bright.

Imagine your inhibitions as an old skin you peel off and throw over your left shoulder.

Breathe out. Imagine your shame as a second old skin that you peel off and throw over your left shoulder.

Breathe out. Imagine your disgust as a third old skin that you peel off and throw over your left shoulder.

Breathe out. See your new skin, pink and luminous.

Breathe out. Open your eyes, seeing the new skin with open eyes.

When you push, you are helping push your baby's head through the birth channel. You will want to open your legs wide and lean back on a firm support. Pushing will feel like pushing out a stool. If you have practiced *Drop of oil* (page 127) when having a hard stool, you will know how helpful it is to visualize the golden oil coating the passage. Here you do the same.

Making sounds is very important; it helps the body push. Don't hold back. You're not there to make others comfortable. They are there to make *you* comfortable and to encourage *you* in every way they can. In chapter 5, you started practicing the sound "beuuu" in *Beuu breathing* (page 127). The deeper, more prolonged, and sustained your sound, the easier and more effective your pushing will be. Make the sound long and low. If "beuu" doesn't work for you, try "moooo" or even "aum" if it is a word you chant regularly. Make it long in the vowels: "auuum." Or find another sound that will open you up.

Remember that breathing out is best for pushing. On the in-breath, arch your belly. Breathe out and push with sustained thrusts so your baby doesn't slip back in. Research shows that slow exhalation pushing at this stage is best.

You will get a lot of encouragement from your support group. In fact, everyone around you is pushing too, lending you their energy and cheering you on. Stay with it. Very soon your baby's head will appear at the mouth of your vagina. This is what is called crowning. If your baby is breech, the presentation will most probably be bottom first or legs first. The baby comes down in a rotating movement.

ROTATING BABY
exercise 98

Close your eyes. Breathe out slowly three times, counting from 3 to 1, seeing the numbers in your mind's eye. See the number 1 as tall, clear, and bright.

See your baby coated in golden sunlit oil, rotating his way down the birth canal.

Breathe out. See his head appearing at the mouth of your vagina or center of the flower.

Breathe out. See the hands of light waiting to receive him. Hear all of nature rejoicing.

Breathe out. Feel the weight of his body as he is placed on your chest.

Breathe out. Look at his face. Smile and welcome him. See him smiling back.

Breathe out. Open your eyes, seeing him with open eyes.

Your baby is spiraling down to the head of the flower at the center of the garden. He comes into the garden of your heart. He will become the central focus of your attention from this moment onward for a long time. Enjoy this extraordinary gift from nature. There is really nothing to compare to the joy of seeing your baby's face for the first time. Time is suspended.

Share that first sight with your partner. Rejoice in your triumph. You and your baby have made it through with the help and support of your partner. You are now wedded together as a family, having shared all the trepidations and hopes of this labor and the nine months preceding it. You are forever linked through love and exultation.

While this is happening, your baby's air passageways—mouth and nostrils—are being suctioned out to enable him to breathe. His first breath will often be accompanied by his first cry. In a minute or so, he turns from blue to a healthy pink. The spirit has entered him, and he is now a full-fledged member of this earthly community his parents live in.

The new practice is to place Baby in his coating of vernix, a thick white cream that protected his skin in the amniotic waters, directly on your chest—your "outer womb"—skin to skin and covered with a blanket to keep him warm. You can ask that the initial newborn assessment be done on your chest.

Within the next five minutes, your partner or someone of your choice will cut the cord, and your baby will begin his life as an independent entity. It is never too early for you to recognize that fact. Mark the moment by whispering in his left ear your special message of welcome. The midwives of the Masai, a Kenyan tribe, are known to whisper into a newborn's ear, "You are responsible for your life as I am for mine!"

If left free to move on your chest, he'll instinctively crawl up to your breast. He may or may not latch on right away. Don't worry. Hold him and smell him and rejoice in his beauty.

Baby will now be taken away, to get checked and tested. He will receive his Apgar score, which tests for heart rate, respiratory effort, muscle tone, reflex irritability, and color. He will be weighed and checked for a good Moro reflex (the infantile reflex of spreading out the arms and pulling them back in response to a sudden sense of loss of support). He will receive erythromycin drops for his eyes and be returned to you.

Stage Three: Delivering the Placenta

Thankfully, your last stage, delivering the placenta, is much simpler than the stages you have just experienced. It happens five to thirty minutes after your baby is born. You will have mild contractions that feel more like menstrual cramps, and you may not even feel them or be aware that the placenta is being delivered. The placenta has been the life support for your baby for nine months. It will now separate from the uterine wall and move down into the vagina, where you will be asked to push it out. Your placenta is taking too long to be expelled? You can do this exercise to push it out, if your doctor agrees.

TO RELEASE THE PLACENTA
exercise 99

Close your eyes. Breathe out slowly three times, counting from 3 to 1, seeing the numbers in your mind's eye. See the number 1 as tall, clear, and bright.

See yourself in a meadow. Smell the grass. Lie down on the thick emerald-green carpet. Let your body sink, feeling the buoyant support of the emerald-green carpet of grass.

Breathe out. See yourself becoming all green, every part of you—your skin, hair, nails, face, eyes, mouth, and genitals.

Breathe out. Sense, see, and feel that you are rolling and undulating like a great serpent of green light. As you undulate, your womb is becoming green too, and it is easily and fluidly releasing the placenta.

Breathe out. See the placenta full of blood and very red against the green grass. See inscribed in the lining of the placenta the upside-down tree that held your baby, bringing it from the sky into the world and into your arms. Thank the placenta.

Breathe out. Standing up, pick up this marvel of nature and go look for the perfect place to bury it. Find some rich soil at the foot of a beautiful tree so that all of its richness will feed the tree and the meadow. Bury it.

Breathe out. Open your eyes.

When the placenta is out, ask to see it. It is a most astonishing organ. It has served your baby as the interface between you and him. It has been his lungs, intestine, kidneys, and bloodstream. It has served to recycle carbon dioxide and waste products back into his mother's blood to be eliminated. On one side, the fetal side, it is white and shiny; on the other side, the side that was attached to the uterine wall, it is bloody. When you look at it, you will see many blood vessels that look like the branches of a tree. The placenta has been your child's tree of life.

Some people might choose to keep the placenta to bury it later on. Perhaps you'll want to plant a tree above where you buried it. This is an ancient tradition followed by many people around the world. The placenta also can be ground up to serve as medicine for baby and you, to help boost your immune systems. Ask your doula; she may know about this. Judith Halleck, one of our original group of birth professionals, does it for her mothers, and you might be able to find someone local who can help you with this.

If you have had an episiotomy or a tear, your doctor or midwife will now stitch it.

WOUND REPAIR (1)
exercise 100

Close your eyes. Breathe out slowly three times, counting from 3 to 1, seeing the numbers in your mind's eye. See the number 1 as tall, clear, and bright.

Imagine that you stretch your arm up toward the sun. Catch a ray of light. Imagine that your doctor or midwife stitches you up with the ray of light. See that the needle also turns into light.

Breathe out. Ask all of your cells to realign within the web of light created by the stitching.

Breathe out. See the cut or tear disappearing in light and the skin smoothing over, until your skin is like new.

Breathe out. Open your eyes.

Your child has come! Your amazement at his beauty knows no bounds. You laugh and cry and feel so happy and grateful that he has come to you. He is a gift beyond any gift you ever imagined receiving. Even if he arrives all scrunched up (which almost never happens if you have done the exercises), you can't take your eyes off him. To you, he is the most marvelous and incredible being you have ever set eyes on. You're falling head over heels in love. So is your partner and everyone else in the room. He is a luminous, utterly pure marvel, just like baby Jesus in the manger. Keep that first precious vision of him—that first touch and smell, that first hearing and tasting of him—in your heart.

When he is born, you will feel reborn. The joy is so exuberantly present that you will feel all your creative juices flow up like a fountain of joy within you. Follow the inspiration of your creativity, which birth helps you tap into in such a direct way. After my son was born, I became a poet. Here is what I wrote about his birth.

TELLING SAM

when I bent down to pull you out of me
your wrinkled arms limp in my big hands
you popped up in the triangle of my legs
I saw you dangling in space
my astonishment burst like a triumphant arc
I lifted you up
you came down on me calm as a Buddha
impressing your weight like a sucking cup
your toes curled in my belly button
your head under my chin, bald as a honeydew
your eyes like wet grapes glistening with memory
you watched the room as if it were thick
you seemed unperturbed by the new light
the voice counting one two three four five
toes, ten fingers, congratulating
your father on your well formed testes
as a hand rolled you over
you lay quiet within the circle of faces
the cord pulsing white and veined as a cow's udder
the silver scissors went skrunch skrunch
your father cutting through
they lifted you away
my flesh dissolved into light particles
running to stretch over you the invisible
membrane

7

First Smiles

I have just three things to teach: simplicity, patience,
compassion. These three are your greatest treasures.

LAO TZU

YOUR LABOR AND delivery are over. You're probably so relieved that you've already forgotten what you just went through. Or you're so exhilarated that you're riding high, both with the success of your birthing and the advent of your child. Your reward lies in the crook of your elbow, happily gurgling and grabbing your finger tightly, her huge eyes gazing deeply into yours (her eyes at birth are nearly the size they'll be when she's fully mature). You may be fatigued and want your partner to take over. Or you may be very talkative—each mom's mood is different—and want to call all your family members and your close friends to tell them Baby has arrived! If you've already chosen a name, you'll say her name, rolling the syllables around your tongue, savoring the moment. If you've asked for full rooming-in, you can start the bonding process right away.

These first moments are very precious. The Hebrew sages called these revelatory falling-in-love moments the "firstlings," which are traditionally offered to God. You offer the firstlings of your apple tree, the firstlings of your ewes, the firstlings of your feelings of joy. Why to

God (call Him mystery or universe, if you prefer)? Because He is the creative force tearing through the veil of the unknown, revealing its first face. He is your co-creator and you are bursting with hallelujahs and gratitude. What experience can ever compare to seeing your baby for the first time? You may even feel like you're going to die of joy. The mystery blows through you as you look at her face. She has your nose but also her father's, your mother's eyes, his father's mouth. She shape-shifts into so many familiar forms and yet is none of them. She is her own beauty, and you are amazed, awed, ravished.

FEELING YOURSELF AFTER BIRTH

Soon after the birth, you'll be surprised at the mixture of joy and discomfort creeping into your awareness. While you delight in your child lying heavy and warm on your chest, you are also feeling wet and swollen between your legs. Your arms encircle her but your muscles ache. She is suckling the watery pre-milk called colostrum, while your insides are crying from thirst and hunger. Your lips hurt where you bit them, your hips feel bruised, your legs throb. Or, if you have had a C-section, you're feeling sore where the incision is and trying to recover from what is, after all, major surgery. You may actually experience a twinge of resentment. Welcome to the joys of parenthood: you are learning your first lesson in what will be a recurring balancing act. You are being trained in the state of mind called paradox, where joys and frustrations are bed partners; you must learn to accommodate both feelings. Your heart goes out to this little being who lies so vulnerable in your arms, yet you long to pee, stretch, deal with the burning in your perineum, and sleep.

Listen to your body. It talks to you about your needs (it will also tell you about your baby's needs—we will talk more about her needs in a moment). Just now you are exhausted, thirsty, and hungry. Be sure to drink as much as you want. Hospitals offer new mothers a traditional glass of orange juice. While drinking—slowly, please—you can fill yourself with the color and sunshine of the orange, the fruit closest in appearance to the sun. It will help relieve your exhaustion. At some point, you'll be taken to your room, where you can ask for food. Maybe your partner has already arranged for your favorite dishes to be delivered. Let him take care of Baby while you eat. Eat slowly and only a little at first. You can always eat more later on. Remember that you've just gone through an incredible marathon. Take it slowly. Then, when you're done, don't forget to suggest that your partner eat too. He has also been through a marathon by supporting you and lending you his energy throughout your labor. Like you, he has dipped deep into his own resources and needs replenishment. Thank him for being there with you. Give him your highest praise. Don't hold back on words of approval and gratitude. He needs to hear from you that you're both in this together and that his part in the pageant is paramount. So many husbands and partners feel left out. It is the Madonna and Child syndrome, with Joseph left out of the picture. Make sure your partner is firmly in the picture. Start now to include him in everything having to do with the new member of your family. Beware from the very first not to become the possessive mother or self-less martyr in your household. You will both be caring for Baby, each one of you in your inimitable and all-important ways.

Don't forget that you can help yourself feel better. Imagery doesn't end when your birthing marathon is over. In fact, I hope it has become an indispensable tool you can always access to heal yourself and your whole family. It is a universal language that has applications across the board. Here are some exercises if you have had a vaginal birth, which will ease the physical pain of the aftermath of birthing.

TO EASE PERINEUM SWELLING
exercise 101

Close your eyes. Breathe out slowly three times, counting from 3 to 1, seeing the numbers in your mind's eye. See the number 1 as tall, clear, and bright.

Imagine taking a large, soft paintbrush, dipping it into indigo-blue ink, and painting your perineum, vulva, and anus indigo blue. See them in that color for one minute.

Breathe out. Ask for the color to remain in that area of your body for seventy-two hours (three days).

Breathe out. Open your eyes, seeing that whole area indigo-blue with open eyes.

Make sure to visualize indigo-blue whenever the discomfort reappears. You may be given a pack of ice to hold between your legs. Both ice and indigo blue are cooling to your flesh, so both will help reduce the discomfort and swelling.

Your muscle aches and bruises also need attending to.

ANGELIC MASSAGE FOR MUSCLE ACHES AND BRUISING
exercise 102

Close your eyes. Breathe out slowly three times, counting from 3 to 1, seeing the numbers in your mind's eye. See the number 1 as tall, clear, and bright.

Imagine warm, sunlit oil being poured over your skin and spread all over you by invisible feather-like fingers. Feel the fingers softly massaging your body all over, including your face and scalp.

Breathe out. See and feel the oil entering through the pores of your skin and pouring down through all your muscles until your body is golden and deeply relaxed.

Breathe out. Feel the feather-like fingers caressing your skin. Then feel the energy field of your body four inches above your body and that of your baby, enveloping you both in a golden, protective cocoon.

Breathe out. Open your eyes.

At some point, you will want to get up. Be careful, as you may be somewhat unsteady at first. You'll want to pee. At first you'll find it's difficult because you're swollen. But continue the icing and the indigo-blue imagery. If you don't get relief, ask to see the doctor or call your midwife. You may have to have a catheter inserted to empty your bladder. But before doing that, try using your imagery. You are now able to invent your own imagery. Here's one imagery exercise in case you're too tired to conjure up your own.

A CATHETER OF LIGHT
exercise 103

Close your eyes. Breathe out slowly three times, counting from 3 to 1, seeing the numbers in your mind's eye. See the number 1 as tall, clear, and bright.

Sing the sound *deee*. Bring it deeply into your belly, seeing how it opens up all your lower openings, including your urethra.

Imagine that you have a transparent pump ending in a long stem. Insert the stem into your wide-open urethra, squeeze the pump, and watch as the yellow urine fills the pump.

Breathe out. When the pump is full, take the stem out of your urethra and pour the urine into Mother Earth, thanking her.

Breathe out. Open your eyes, feeling relieved.

How to sleep after such excitement? Can you? Both you and your baby need sleep. Your newborn will need as much as sixteen hours' sleep a day but will awaken to feed every two to four hours, which disrupts your sleep pattern. Your partner is either falling asleep on the cot provided by the hospital or has gone home. If you've had a home birth, just cuddle up together, the three of you, and go to sleep. If your excitement keeps you awake, it may be that your adrenals are still secreting noradrenaline, the fight-or-flight hormone that is at its peak release during the final contractions before delivery. The effect of this adrenal release is to ensure that both you and your baby are wide awake and alert at the time of delivery. The open-eyed look and dilated pupils of your baby are signs of adrenal release. In your case, the adrenal release may have been so intense as to keep you awake and overexcited when everyone else and your baby are already fast asleep.

ADRENAL HANDLES
exercise 104

Close your eyes. Breathe out slowly three times, counting from 3 to 1, seeing the numbers in your mind's eye. See the number 1 as tall, clear, and bright.

See your adrenal glands as two oblong shapes resembling boomerangs. Imagine them as two handles.

Breathe out. Lift your hands up toward the sun. Fill them with rainbow colors from the prism of sunlight you hold in your hands.

Breathe out. Bring your hands down and take hold of the two adrenal glands.

Breathe out. Caress and soothe them from top to bottom, letting the rainbow lights penetrate them. Do this three times from top to bottom, caressing, warming, bringing light into those two oblong handles that are your adrenals. Pay attention to the color or colors that remain when you have done this.

Breathe out. Sense the flow of hormones from your adrenals streaming through your whole body as colored light. What color do you see? How does your body feel now?

Breathe out. Open your eyes.

BONDING WITH YOUR BABY

Taking care of your needs first may feel strange to you. But when the flight attendant on a plane reviews safety procedures, she tells you to put on your oxygen mask first before adjusting your child's mask. It is the same here. If you're clean, refreshed, and comfortable—and don't hesitate to ask for help from your close ones, as this is not a time for you to be worrying about house chores or food—you'll be more attentive to your baby. You want those first hours to be entirely rosy hued. Think of the nativity scene, so peaceful and filled with light. All eyes are turned toward baby Jesus in his cradle of hay. With the birth of your baby, you have been flooded with oxytocin, a hormone that is often called the love hormone. It was released at the time of intercourse when Baby was conceived, and again at her birth when oxytocin helped your uterus to contract and expel the fetus. You are flooded with it right now.

BONDING WITH YOUR NEWBORN
exercise 105

Breathe out a light smoke and with it all that disturbs you, pains you, obscures you. With the inhalation, breathe in the blue-gold light from the sky.

See and feel this blue-gold light entering in your nostrils, flowing down into your throat.

See it as a great river of light flowing down your back, into your legs, feet, toes. See the light emanating from each toe as a long, blue-gold antenna.

Now see this river of light travel up your legs to your pelvic region, filling it with light and creating a blue-gold space inside your uterus.

Breathe out. From your uterus, cast a blue-gold net over your baby. Feel and see your baby bathed in the warmth of this healing light and send your love through every strand of light. See and feel how you are one, still connected, as you were when your baby was inside you. See and feel how your baby responds.

Breathe out. The river of light continues to rise up into your chest and flow in and out of the four chambers of your heart until your heart becomes a great glowing lamp.

See the light flow up to your shoulders and down into your arms, hands, and fingers, stretching out of your fingers like long antennae of light. Hold your baby in the crook of your left elbow, near your great glowing heart. See and feel how your baby is being bathed in love and soothing blue-gold light. Feel this connection in all of your body, mind, heart, and soul.

Breathe out. Open your eyes, seeing the connection with open eyes.

This is your basic exercise for always keeping engaged with your newborn. You will recognize it as a variation on the *Blue vase* exercise (page 100) you practiced throughout your pregnancy. Imagine the blue-gold mesh stretching out over your baby when you have to be apart. While physically separated from you, your baby will continue to experience your comforting presence and feel safe.

Newborns are particularly aware of dreamfields, as they spend around sixteen hours a day sleeping and more than eight hours in active REM (rapid eye movement) dreaming. You can confidently communicate with them through "the airways." You've been doing just that for the last nine months, and you've been able to verify its efficacy. You will learn a lot about this means of communication as you grow in your parenting skills. It's called intuition, the invisible telephone. You "know" how your child feels even at a distance. But what most people don't realize is that you can also "send" support and love via the same airways through which you receive. It's done through images. Your child will "know" what messages you are sending her. You will have an instantaneous effect on her moods, comfort, and sense of safety.

If, for some reason—a medical issue, hospital regulations, or the need for rest—your baby is not with you but in the common nursery, you will want to actively practice seeing the blue-gold net enveloping her so you can psychically keep her close. If baby was born early and is in the neonatal room, visualize her undeveloped organs growing perfectly. See and sense your hands of light touching her, the net of light enveloping her.

While it is not always possible to keep baby physically close to you (and you shouldn't feel bad or guilty about what can't be helped or about needing to get some well-earned rest), research clearly shows that baby benefits most from staying close to you, especially in those first hours and days after birth. She wants to be with you, as hypnotic regressions to the birth and aftermath show. Again and again in those sessions, the regressed adults hone in on their great need and longing to be with Mom. If not with you, Baby will want to be with her father, whose presence, research also proves, she recognizes right from the start.

NEWBORN TALENTS

For a long time, doctors and researchers were under the impression that newborns started as simple creatures with no feelings, no brains to speak of, no true awareness. Jean Piaget, the Swiss psychologist, called them "solipsistic," meaning that in the first weeks of their life, newborns showed no interest in their environment. Until recently, experts thought that what happened in the first moments and weeks of a child's life wasn't particularly significant for its future development. This viewpoint affected everything from parking babies away from their mothers in hospital nurseries to not offering pain management; since newborns were supposed to be largely unconscious, it followed that they wouldn't feel pain. Thanks to the wealth of research being done today on neonates, doctors and experts have changed their minds. They now recognize what mothers, fathers, grandparents, and relatives have known all along: Baby is aware, present, and in need of the attention of her choice people from the moment of her birth.

That the first four hours following birth are crucial is dramatically demonstrated with rats, dogs, sheep, and goats. Take the newborn animal away from its mother and the mother will refuse to interact with its newborn when it is returned hours later. Allow the newborn to remain in Mom's company during those crucial first hours and she'll accept her baby back and nurture it following separation, even when the separation time is prolonged. Likewise, early contact between human babies and their mothers "makes a significant difference in health, growth, and learning," says psychologist David Chamberlain. Those newborns gain weight more rapidly; show greater resilience, motor coordination, and muscle control sooner; test consistently higher in language skills and on IQ scores at two years old; and are more secure, trusting, and confident children overall. "All subsequent interactions are enriched," says Chamberlain, by giving your full and undivided attention to your newborn at birth.

Mothers, too, are more secure, calm, and confident in handling their babies when they have been able to bond in those early hours.

Baby is not "a pound of flesh"; Baby is a person! She has a mind far more advanced than her brain or body, and a personality that is easily observable for the first eight days of her life. After that, baby fat will mask her true face and you won't see it reappearing until she's fully mature, around early adulthood. In the same way that doctors can measure the length of the baby's foot and calculate how tall she'll be, you can read her face and know what kind of a person she has all the marks of becoming.

Already at birth, your newborn is an amazingly complex and highly developed being. She instinctively knows how to use all her senses to gravitate toward you, her mother. She scans faces in the delivery room until she locates yours and locks on, even though she has never before laid eyes on you (did she dream your face in the womb?). She contentedly gazes into your eyes, pouring that invisible and potent nectar called love from her eyes to yours and hungrily taking in love from yours. She naturally cuddles up to your particular curves and turns her mouth toward your breast (research shows that she is not as comfortable adapting her body to other bodies and their curves). She knows, from smell, which is your milk and can distinguish it from the start from all other mothers' milk.

Your newborn also recognizes your voice. She has been listening to it in the womb for nine months. She may actually be picking up the vibrations of your voice not only with her ear but through her skin, the largest sense organ in the body. The skin, says Alfred Tomatis, the French hearing specialist, has similar sensory cells to the Corti cells that populate the ear. While the baby listens with her ears, she also *feels* your sounds from your skin that vibrates as you speak. This is why placing your newborn skin to skin on your chest immediately after birth has so many benefits. With this skin-to-skin contact, she also gets to sample your smell, your touch, and your temperature. In fact, she learns to regulate her temperature as well as her heart rate, breathing, hormone levels, and enzyme production, all from cuddling with Mom. It takes infants who aren't in their mother's company much longer to learn to regulate.

SKIN TO SKIN
exercise 106

Close your eyes. Breathe out slowly three times, counting from 3 to 1, seeing the numbers in your mind's eye. See the number 1 as tall, clear, and bright.

Breathe out. Sense, see, and feel that every cell of your skin is an eye.

Breathe out. Sense, see, and feel that every cell in your skin is an ear.

Breathe out. Look at and listen to your baby through your skin. What do you experience, see, and learn?

Breathe out. Smell the different scents emanating from your baby. How does this change your touch as you caress your baby? How does it change your baby? What do you feel in your own body and skin? Describe it.

Breathe out. Open your eyes.

While you are learning about your baby from your skin contact and through all your senses, she is using her senses to learn about you. From the moment she's born, Baby learns. She was learning in the womb. Now she does it through her interaction with the people who surround her. Since your baby's primary relationship is with you, she learns mainly through "dialoguing" with you. She is already familiar with your voice, your rhythms, your smells, your taste; she recognizes your face. She responds to your caresses, smiles, and words and challenges you back through her cries, smiles, whistles, and hoots. She doesn't have words, but she does possess expressions, body movements, and sounds. This is her way of informing you and calling you forth. Already in your first encounter, she searches and finds you, cuddles up to you, looks up at you.

SKY IN THE EYES
exercise 107

Close your eyes. Breathe out slowly three times, counting from 3 to 1, seeing the numbers in your mind's eye. See the number 1 as tall, clear, and bright.

Looking into your baby's eyes, see and feel how the great unknown from whence your baby comes is soft and limitless like the sky.

Allow yourself to go into the sky of her eyes, to feel its soft, limitless space.

Breathe out. Sense all the changes in your body.

Slowly return to your physical sensations, calling your baby by name.

What do you see happening?

Breathe out. Open your eyes.

These first moments together determine many factors about your baby's future. Call these the firstlings of relationship. Her first impressions leave a lasting imprint, for good or bad, upon your baby's subconscious. She has never been apart from you. She needs the familiarity of your presence and rhythms to be able to integrate all her new experiences. She needs your arms around her to safeguard her from space, that vast unknown. She needs time in a safe environment to adjust to the great changes birth has wrought in her world. You have been talking, touching, smelling, tasting, and listening to her since conception. Now that she is here in the flesh—complete with all her body, brain, and inner parts—you must anchor her in her embodiment. Your touch, your warmth, your smell, your voice, your love are her recognizable signposts in this brave new world she has ventured into.

BABY'S NAME—THE SOUND OF LOVE
exercise 108

Close your eyes. Breathe out slowly three times, counting from 3 to 1, seeing the numbers in your mind's eye. See the number 1 as tall, clear, and bright.

Look into your baby's eyes and call her forth by calling her name. How does your baby respond?

Breathe out. Call out the sound of your baby's name again and hear it as you linger over the syllables.

Breathe out. Calling out your baby's name a third time, hear it as the sound of love. What images, colors, sensations, and feelings do you have?

Breathe out. Open your eyes.

TAKING CARE OF BABY

All your imagery has been training you in how to handle your baby. Every gesture, unbeknownst to you, starts with an image. Becoming aware of that desire-image, being conscious of it, transforms every gesture you make into a subtle, caring movement. The image starts with a flash of light and evolves into a fluid form, generating the nervous impulse that becomes the physical movement, ending at, say, touching your baby's plump little legs or soft cheek.

Enter the physical component. Will the lessons of caring that you practiced through imagery during your pregnancy be manifested in real life? Remember that for nine months your baby was in a contained environment, the walls of the amniotic sac anchoring her. When she comes into your hands, don't be afraid to hold her firmly. She needs to learn from your hands that she is safe. Nervous or hesitant gestures will confuse her. Holding her too tightly will hurt or threaten her.

Hands talk. They talk through the desire-image, whether it is the love-image or the fear-image. Babies can read your hands. Their minds are attuned to information through their right brain, their left brain having yet to acquire the words to distinguish what is happening to them. But have no doubt that they feel and "know" what is happening to them. It is a fact, confirmed by many studies, that infants need loving touch. Orphans in foundling homes and preemies isolated in incubators have been seen to wither and die for lack of stroking. Today, orphanages and hospitals have a policy of stroking and massaging every three hours. Preemies also are touched and caressed at regular intervals and, when possible, held by their parents.

HAND HOLDING
exercise 109

Close your eyes. Breathe out slowly three times, counting from 3 to 1, seeing the numbers in your mind's eye. See the number 1 as tall, clear, and bright.

As you pick your baby up, sense, see, and feel the palms of your hands holding her.

Breathe out. Sense how the palms of your hands speak to your baby. If you are not satisfied with how they are speaking to your baby, make the necessary changes.

Breathe out. Sense how your baby speaks to you through the palms of your hands. What is changing between you and your baby?

Breath out. Open your eyes.

As Baby learns, she is also teaching you. The first thing she teaches you is to respond instead of react, which is the difference between respecting the other's feelings and being indifferent or callous toward their needs. Baby will let you know. She has no restraints and no shame. She will cry if your grip is too tight or whimper if your hands are hesitant or nervous. She will let you know if your hands are rough or insensitive or tentative. If you're not responding, she'll cry more. If you react to her crying by getting angry with her, she'll up the ante. She has no way of tempering or transmuting her emotions. You do. The Divine or Mystery has given her to you so that, softened by love, you will learn ways of quieting your impulses and transforming your emotions. Baby teaches you how to forget yourself. She teaches you how to put yourself in her place, to feel what she feels, to have empathy. Having the imagination to become the other for a moment is what love is. With Baby, you learn unconditional love.

PUTTING YOURSELF IN BABY'S PLACE
exercise 110

Close your eyes. Breathe out slowly three times, counting from 3 to 1, seeing the numbers in your mind's eye. See the number 1 as tall, clear, and bright.

See yourself once again as a baby.

Sense, see, and feel, like a baby, being wet for a long time.

Breathe out. Being hungry for a long time.

Breathe out. Being left alone for a long time.

Breathe out. Sense, see, and feel, like a baby, being rocked and sung to.

Breathe out. Open your eyes.

Knowing what your baby feels will enable you to respond to her needs in an attuned and caring manner. The best way to do this is by using your imagination: put yourself geographically as well as sizewise and agewise in her place and, for a moment, become her. Trust what you feel when switching places with her. You can test the accuracy of your images when you address her needs as you felt them from switching places. If you get the result you expected, you have verified that you truly "know" what she feels.

WHAT DOES BABY'S SKIN NEED?
exercise III

Close your eyes. Breathe out slowly three times, counting from 3 to 1, seeing the numbers in your mind's eye. See the number 1 as tall, clear, and bright.

Sense and see yourself rocking your baby.

Breathe out. Become the baby in your arms. Sense, see, and smell your mother; cuddle up to her.

Breathe out. Sense and feel what your skin needs from your mother.

Breathe out. Is there a part of your body that needs more touch and comfort?

Breathe out. Returning to your adult perspective, how do you change what you are doing with your baby? How does she respond?

Breathe out. Open your eyes.

For years, until I was in my thirties, I felt a gaping hole in the small of my neck. My skin there was always cold. With a desperation I couldn't explain even to myself, I longed for a hand to hold up the back of my neck and head. I was born in England at the end of World War II. My mother already had a one-year-old son. She had no milk to breast-feed and was herself on a starvation diet. She probably kept me in my cradle most of the time, if only to keep me warm. I cried a lot. Deprivation comes not only from food but also from other senses. It was the reassuring and life-giving contact with the crook of her elbow that I was missing and that accounted for my cold neck.

Babies teach us simplicity. They teach us how to return to the basics, how to sense the other, how to intuit what they need. They teach us all over again the language of the body. For that, we must be willing to listen patiently, to respond compassionately. If we have wanted a baby only to serve our own needs, we're going to be rudely awakened. Baby is an inestimable gift, but we must learn to deserve it.

HATCHING
exercise 112

Close your eyes. Breathe out slowly three times, counting from 3 to 1, seeing the numbers in your mind's eye. See the number 1 as tall, clear, and bright.

Imagine that you are holding an egg and warming it in the palms of your hands. Be very careful how you hold the egg: don't hold it too tight, or it might break; don't hold it too loosely, or it might slip out of your hands.

Breathe out. Put all of your energy and love into your hands to warm the egg. Be patient and wait until you feel movement inside the egg. You have to be very careful when the egg moves and then breaks open. What are you feeling?

Breathe out. You are still holding the egg as the chick comes out of its shell.

Breathe out. Let go of the eggshell. Adjust your hands to hold the newborn chick. What are you feeling when you hold it?

Watch as it grows. What are you feeling now?

Do not put the chick down until it is ready to go exploring on its own.

Breathe out. Open your eyes.

Babies are physically helpless but mentally very much alert and eager to learn. They use their eyes to scan everything in sight. They are particularly interested in your face, your smiles, your sounds, your gestures, and those of their father or older siblings. From the very first day, they match their movements to the rhythm of your movements and sounds. Like a finely tuned instrument, they imitate what they see and hear. Baby is your clear mirror. Baby calls forth your very best from within you. Offer your baby your joy, your hope, your happiness. And if you cannot do so, at least offer your baby your love.

BABY AS MIRROR
exercise 113

Close your eyes. Breathe out slowly three times, counting from 3 to 1, seeing the numbers in your mind's eye. See the number 1 as tall, clear, and bright.

Seeing your baby, experience her purity and newness as the descent of the Divine or Mystery into your daily life.

Breathe out. See her watching you and imitating everything you do. How does this affect your gestures, your mood?

Breathe out. Recognize that she is the mirror reflecting back to you who you are. How do you live up to that responsibility?

Breathe out. Open your eyes.

If this is difficult or painful for you, don't worry. Accept your feelings, whatever they are. Having self-compassion is always the first step toward healing yourself. We will be dealing with guilt, resentment, vulnerability, and overall difficulties and fears of motherhood further along.

BREAST-FEEDING

After the birth of your baby, the hormones you need for breast-feeding are best stimulated by skin-to-skin contact with her. Holding her, caressing her, gazing into her eyes, are some of the ways in which oxytocin, the love hormone, is released. In chapter 6, we saw that oxytocin levels peak at birth, enabling the uterus to expel the placenta. After birth, the hormone is a powerful relaxant, bringing heart rate and blood pressure down, reducing pain and anxiety, and encouraging you to get close, snuggle up, and embrace your baby. It will not serve you to think that love is simply a chemical reaction. Perhaps your feelings of love also encourage the release of the hormone. There is no separation between body and mind. Your mothering instinct is at the same time a feeling and a hormone release.

As you relax, oxytocin triggers your milk ejection reflex (also called the let-down reflex) by inducing the breast muscle contractions that squeeze out your milk. Your body also produces beta-endorphins, pain blockers that trigger the release of prolactin, the third hormone you need for lactation. Prolactin causes your breast glands to produce colostrum, your pre-milk, followed three days later by your milk. Release of these three hormones has a cascading effect on your ability to breast-feed. Nature in her wisdom has devised the best way for your baby to get what she needs. So it makes sense to follow nature and allow your baby to breast-feed as soon after birth as possible.

As I mentioned before, colostrum is a yellowish watery substance that contains an impressive array of antibodies and proteins to protect and stimulate your baby's immune system and gut. It also acts as a mild laxative to help your baby pass her first stool (meconium) and clear the bilirubin, a waste product of dead red cells that, if retained by the liver, could result in jaundice.

If Baby is placed belly down on your chest, she will inch herself up to your breast and latch on instinctively. She will find her own way. You don't need to coax her or change positions. Sitting up won't make your milk flow any better because gravity is not necessary for milk to flow. All you need is suction. So the best position for breast-feeding her is whatever position best suits you and Baby.

Whatever the size of their breasts, all mothers can breast-feed. By touching the baby's chin, you coax her to open her mouth wide and encircle the whole areola of your breast with her lips. You don't want her to just hold on to your nipple. If your nipples are flat or inverted, however, your baby will have a harder time suckling, even if the position of her lips is good. In her efforts to latch on, her gums can squeeze and irritate your areola. Don't wait for this to happen, as your anxiety and frustration can exacerbate your emotional vulnerability after giving birth. Don't start feeling afraid that your baby will go hungry and that you'll turn out to be an inadequate mother. Before guilt and resentment of the helpless little being in your arms set in, remember to sweep those emotions off to the left (*Sweep the porch,* page 75) and start practicing the next exercise. You can do it before nursing, but also in the first days of nursing, as many times as you like. This will stimulate your nipple to become erect as soon as baby indicates it's time for her feeding.

TURNING NIPPLES INSIDE OUT
exercise 114

Close your eyes. Breathe out slowly three times, counting from 3 to 1, seeing the numbers in your mind's eye. See the number 1 as tall, clear, and bright.

Imagine that you are in a meadow on a bright, clear day. Look up at the sun.

Stretch your arms up toward the sun. Feel them elongating until your hands feels warm, then filled with light.

Breathe out. Point an index finger toward the sun and see the light touching it so that the tip of your finger shines like a star.

Breathe out. Bring your arms back down to their normal size.

Breathe out. See yourself in a mirror naked from the waist up. With your hands of light, massage your left breast, moving from the periphery toward the nipple.

Breathe out. Have your hands of light go into your breast. Use your fingers of light to massage the inside of your areola and nipple. Pay attention to all the sensations in your nipple and breast.

Breathe out. Sense and see your lit index finger pushing your nipple out from the inside.

Breathe out. Take your hands out of your breast. Still in front of the mirror, see your hands of light first squeezing the areola, then stretching it out. See your nipple in the mirror. How does it look and feel now?

Breathe out. Repeat the exercise for the other breast.

Breathe out. See both your breasts in the mirror. See your nipples erect.

Breathe out. Open your eyes, sensing your erect nipples with open eyes.

If you are still having difficulty breast-feeding, ask for help from the nurses at the hospital or from your midwife. A lactating consultant can be sent to see you and the baby. You will do better if you let go of your spiraling negative thoughts and emotions. Instead, sink back into your body and into feeling your baby's body. After sweeping your emotions to the left, surround yourself and your baby in a protective cocoon (*The cocoon of light,* page 74) Then, remembering that your breathing changes when you're agitated, learn to always approach your baby in a quiet state. Remember to enter the "zone"—the timeless, light-filled space of love.

TIMELESS BUBBLE
exercise 115

Close your eyes. Breathe out slowly three times, counting from 3 to 1, seeing the numbers in your mind's eye. See the number 1 as tall, clear, and bright.

See, feel, and sense time slowing down as you approach your baby. Sense your footsteps slowing down more and more until you are moving in slow motion.

Breathe out. See time becoming a drop of light between you and your baby. See the drop of light expanding to encompass both of you, and feel yourself in this timeless bubble of communion.

Breathe out. Step back, seeing the expanded light return to just a drop of light, then expand again to become a pulsing rhythmic arc of light between the two of you.

Breathe out. Move back into the fast pace of your daily work life while still being connected through the pulsing arc of light.

Breathe out. Do this three times.

Breathe out. Open your eyes.

Whatever your difficulties, don't give up on breast-feeding your baby the colostrum. For centuries, colostrum was considered impure for Baby to drink. Now that scientific studies have determined its components, we know that colostrum is valuable and will give your baby a great boost. In the first few days of her life, Baby drinks at most the equivalent of a thimbleful of colostrum, so there is not much yet to do in the way of breast-feeding except to practice and make sure your baby gets that thimbleful.

After two or three days of disgorging colostrum, your breasts produce milk. The moment is called engorgement, and with the surplus of milk and hormones, your breasts will swell to double their size. It will hurt a bit, but think of it as a great natural joke. I remember a father looking at his wife's engorged breasts and exclaiming, "I wish you would do that for me!" In a day or two, the swelling will subside and you'll be more comfortable, provided you empty both breasts, alternating between breasts at each feeding.

Don't let stress inhibit the let-down; the stress hormone adrenaline will stop the milk flow. Know that your baby is not going to starve. Babies generally lose weight the first week, only to regain it the second. But if you hold your baby kangaroo-fashion near your skin at all times, she probably won't lose any weight.

Again, the secret to easy breast-feeding is trust. Trust your body and your baby's body. Keep your baby close to you and surrender to your body's instincts. Relaxation and loving contentment will follow. One way to hold your baby close is in a baby sling, which is very comfortable for both baby and you. She can breast-feed in the sling while you continue doing whatever you're doing.

BABY SMILES AND BABY CRIES

Smiles and cries are Baby's way of communicating.

We love her smiles, and we generally respond by smiling back. At birth and for the next six weeks, you may notice that her smiles are not focused—they don't quite reach up to her eyes. This may be due to a lack of facial muscle development. At six weeks, she will begin to smile properly in response to whatever tickling, cooing, cuddling, or smiling you engage in. The more you smile at her, the more she'll smile back. A smiley baby is one who has been smiled at a lot. Your baby is so attuned to you that your moods will invariably affect hers. She feels everything you feel. If you show her a blank or angry face, she'll turn away or cry. If you smile at her, she'll be happy.

COLOR OF YOUR MOOD
exercise 116

Close your eyes. Breathe out slowly three times, counting from 3 to 1, seeing the numbers in your mind's eye. See the number 1 as tall, clear, and bright.

See, feel, and recognize the color of your mood as you pick up your baby. When you have identified the color, if you don't like it, sweep the color out of your body to the left.

Breathe out. Find the color you like, the color that makes you feel good. See it moving throughout your body and filling it up. What do you feel now?

Breathe out. See the effect this has on your child.

Breathe out. Open your eyes.

Babies cry when they sense your bad moods, when they're uncomfortable, when they need something, when they're bored, and when they hurt. Babies have many different types of cries. You will soon learn to recognize what each one of your baby's cries means.

Why is the sound of a crying baby so difficult for us to handle? Although your breathing accelerates when you hear your baby cry, your breathing rate remains slower than the rhythm of her cries. Nature, in her wisdom, has devised this exquisite form of irritation as a survival mechanism. By crying, your baby is signaling that she needs you *now*. Your discomfort will propel you toward her. Don't make her wait out of a thwarted desire to discipline or get control over her. At this age, your baby is helpless to move on her own or take care of her physical needs. It would be cruel to ignore her.

SIGHING SOFTLY, *AAAH*
exercise 117

Close your eyes. Breathe out slowly three times, counting from 3 to 1, seeing the numbers in your mind's eye. See the number 1 as tall, clear, and bright.

Hear your baby crying. Sense how the rhythm of your baby's crying is faster than your own breathing. What do you feel?

Breathe out. Breathe in the blue-gold light from the sky into your mouth.

Sighing softly, *aaah,* send the blue-gold light to envelop your baby.

Do it again. What other sound or word do you want to use when sighing softly?

Breathe out. Open your eyes.

If your pediatrician is of the old school, he'll recommend that you let the baby cry. Don't listen to your pediatrician without first thinking it through. You have signed up to take care of Baby. As long as she isn't able to propel herself around and meet her own needs, she needs you.

There will be time enough later on to discipline your child and help her develop self-soothing skills.

Even though you now understand what is irritating you when your baby cries, you may still feel frustrated. I remember a young mother who came into my office and cried, "I'm so angry with him!" I thought she meant her husband. But she was angry with her infant son for crying. Why was he crying? Because he was hungry. "Do you give him his bottle at the same time every day?" I asked (she wasn't breast-feeding). "Well, no, I wait until he lets me know he's hungry!" Some people waste time being angry rather than taking care of what needs to be done.

TICK TOCK
exercise 118

Close your eyes. Breathe out slowly three times, counting from 3 to 1, seeing the numbers in your mind's eye. See the number 1 as tall, clear, and bright.

Hear a doorbell ringing. Stop the sound.

Breathe out. Hear your baby crying. Sense and feel what is happening in your body. Stop the sound.

Breathe out. Hear the tick tock, tick tock of a metronome. What is happening to you and to your baby?

Breathe out. Open your eyes.

The metronome will remind baby of the sound of your heartbeats that rocked her in your womb. Holding Baby near your heart will help quiet her. This is why it's intuitive to hold her on your left side. According to psychologist and researcher Lee Salk, most "Madonna and Child" paintings have the infant Jesus lying on his mother's left side.

HEART COHERENCE
exercise 119

Close your eyes. Breathe out slowly three times, counting from 3 to 1, seeing the numbers in your mind's eye. See the number 1 as tall, clear, and bright.

Hold your baby in your left arm.

Breathe out. Go down into the secret chamber at the center of your heart. Listen to your baby's heartbeats through your own heartbeats.

What is happening to the rhythm of your two hearts?

Breathe out. Wait and listen until both hearts beat synchronously. What changes? How are you relating to your baby now?

Breathe out. Open your eyes.

Your heart will beat most calmly and regularly when you allow it to be filled with gratitude and joy for your baby, whose head lies on your bosom near your heart and whose eyes look up at you adoringly.

GRATITUDE (2)

exercise 120

Close your eyes. Breathe out slowly three times, counting from 3 to 1, seeing the numbers in your mind's eye. See the number 1 as tall, clear, and bright.

Sense, see, and feel where your child has come from.

Breathe out. Sense and feel the mystery.

Breathe out. See and feel that your child is a gift from sovereign life to your life. Feel all the gratitude that a gift brings with it.

Breathe out. See your gratitude as a color that emanates from your heart and spreads throughout your body.

Breathe out. See it spreading beyond your skin, enveloping your baby, spreading out to all forms of life in this beautiful world of ours—earth, plants, animals, water, sky.

Breathe out. See and feel this gratitude for all life returning to envelop and sustain your baby. See your baby growing up perfectly.

Breathe out. Open your eyes, feeling and seeing your perfect baby with open eyes.

TAKING CARE OF YOU

We've touched on this idea of self-care at every stage of the mothering journey. But in this stage self-care can be incredibly challenging. First-time parents are always surprised by how much work a newborn requires. Not only must you hold and rock her, you'll need to wash her, change her diapers regularly, and feed her every couple of hours for the first months. Luckily, if you're breast-feeding, you won't have to prepare, heat, and sterilize baby bottles.

Your baby is going to let you know when she's hungry, wet, cold, uncomfortable, in pain, or bored. If you're always carrying her kangaroo-style in a sling, you'll know what she needs before she cries, and you can prevent the crying by taking care of her needs before she acts up.

The most difficult thing to deal with is sleep deprivation. Unfortunately, there's no way around it. Your sleep hours are going to be choppy—you won't be getting more than two to three hours of sleep at a stretch, especially if you have to get up to take care of Baby. You will lose less sleep if she sleeps with you. Apart from the fact that skin-to-skin contact with your baby is so beneficial, sleeping with your baby allows you to feed her while you're both half asleep. Talk to your partner, as this is something you must both agree on. If you're worried that you may roll over her in your sleep, know that the likelihood is practically nonexistent. Both you and your partner are so attuned to her presence that you will wake up before that can happen.

Sleep deprivation can be difficult to deal with and even debilitating. Some people get teary and emotional when they don't get enough sleep. You already know of one exercise that boosts energy, *Blue vase* (page 100). Here is another that puts you in the dream state for a moment so that, in the time it takes you to do the exercise, you get the benefits of a short nap.

SLEEP CRADLE
exercise 121

Close your eyes. Breathe out slowly three times, counting from 3 to 1, seeing the numbers in your mind's eye. See the number 1 as tall, clear, and bright.

Imagine that you are walking on a white sand beach. Find a place where the sand is soft and very white. Lie down in the sand and dig yourself a cradle of sand.

Breathe out. Feel the sun warming your front and the grains of sand warming your back. Rest in your cocoon of sunlight, listening to the lapping of the waves rocking you to sleep. Feel yourself sinking into a deep sleep.

Breathe out. See yourself having a dream of sunlight and sand, hearing the sounds of lapping waves in the ocean. See what else is happening in your dream.

Breathe out. In your dream, see yourself falling asleep and having a dream of sunlight and sand, hearing the sounds of lapping waves in the ocean.

Breathe out. Again, see yourself falling asleep and having a dream of sunlight and sand, hearing the sounds of lapping waves in the ocean.

Breathe out. Feel yourself rising through the three layers of dream and awakening in the cradle of sand on the white sand beach as you hear the lapping of the waves.

Breathe out. Stand up and stretch, feeling the sun, the warm breeze, the cool spray of the ocean. Look at the different blues of the ocean and the sky.

Breathe out. Walk away from the beach, feeling refreshed and energized.

Breathe out. Open your eyes.

Plunging deep into yourself will feel like having a nice rest. By tapping into the dream state, you give your body the pause and refreshment it needs. Practice *Blue vase* (page 100) to get a boost of energy. Practice *Sleep cradle* to catch up on your sleep.

BABY BLUES AND FEARS OF MOTHERHOOD

If you are still feeling tired, irritable, and weepy after having practiced these exercises, you could have the baby blues. This is a condition that affects 60 to 80 percent of women, starting a few days after birth or any time during the first year of motherhood. One of the causes is that estrogen and progesterone levels drop significantly after childbirth, affecting your mood and outlook on life. From a great emotional high, you are suddenly plunged into the pits. Irritability, anxiety, sadness, restlessness, disturbed sleep, and altered eating patterns contribute to the anticlimactic feelings you may have after a highly expected event. The feelings that may surface include disappointment at yourself for not having had the birth you wanted, or at your baby, who doesn't look half as pretty as you'd expected; loss of a comfortable closeness with your partner; resentment that all the attention that was centered on you when you were pregnant has suddenly shifted to Baby; and fear of motherhood.

From exhaustion to guilt is a short road you want to avoid. Generally, baby blues have no one definable cause. Your body needs time to recover and to adjust, a luxury you may not have. As I mentioned before, asking your mother, family member, friend, or even hired help to come in to handle household chores will give you the time you need to recover. In the Netherlands, new mothers are sent a postpartum maternity helper to cook for, clean, and take care of the older kids to reduce the chances of the baby blues becoming a full-fledged postpartum depression. Getting back into your body is an important step in recovering your bearings.

GROUNDING
exercise 122

Close your eyes. Breathe out slowly three times, counting from 3 to 1, seeing the numbers in your mind's eye. See the number 1 as tall, clear, and bright.

Imagine that you are walking deep into an orchard. Listen to your footsteps and hear the sounds of nature.

Breathe out. You come upon a clearing where there are many different kinds of trees. Look around and choose the tree that attracts you the most.

Breathe out. Go and put your arms around the trunk of the tree, feet sinking into the ground. Feel your toes becoming long roots.

Breathe out. Put your left ear to the tree and listen to what the tree says or sounds out.

Breathe out. Become one with your tree. Be the roots, the trunk, the branches, the leaves. Feel each and every part of your tree at the same time. See and feel the sap rising until you feel completely energized and restored.

Breathe out. Step away from the tree. What do you look and feel like now? What does your tree look like?

Breathe out. If you are not pleased with the way your tree looks now, imagine going to a stream nearby, filling a can with water, and returning to water your tree. How does your tree look now? Do this until you are satisfied.

Breathe out. Open your eyes.

While exhaustion and emotional lows are best met by having housekeeping help, fear of motherhood is addressed by having experienced women around you: mothers, doulas, or nurses. Let them help you over the hurdles of familiarizing yourself with your newborn and all that she requires of you. You may not have realized what having a child entails. If you are a perfectionist, you may feel overwhelmed by the commitment and responsibility required. It's difficult to take care of an infant if you still feel like a child who needs care yourself. No wonder you're feeling weepy most of the time.

COMFORTING THE CHILD INSIDE
exercise 123

Close your eyes. Breathe out slowly three times, counting from 3 to 1, seeing the numbers in your mind's eye. See the number 1 as tall, clear, and bright.

Sense, see, and hear yourself as a child crying. See what is happening, in what location, and who, if anyone, is with you.

Breathe out. Take her in your arms and comfort her, telling her that you are going to take care of her from now on.

Breathe out. Take her out to play in the meadow. Tell her she's free to play and to grow.

Breathe out. When she's grown, embrace her again, holding her close until you merge.

Breathe out. Open your eyes.

If you suffer from a more acute case of the baby blues, you may also suffer from PMS (short for premenstrual syndrome), a predictable pattern of emotional and physical symptoms that some women invariably experience before and during their menses, severely enough to disrupt their normal activities. These symptoms vary from woman to woman and reappear with the baby blues. It is important for you to know and hold on to the fact that your sadness is hormone related and has no "real" cause. Don't try to find causes to explain away your blues; this would only make matters worse.

On the other hand, you are probably at risk for postpartum depression if rest and help don't work, you have difficulty concentrating, you are losing interest in Baby and those around you, and you have fantasies of harming yourself or your baby. PPD is a severe condition that requires professional help. Many factors can predispose you to PPD, among them a prior history of depression, a stressful life situation (relationship, finance, job), and heredity. Here is a simple exercise to clear the first signs of PPD or simply a bad case of the baby blues.

MIRROR BLUES
exercise 124

Close your eyes. Breathe out slowly three times, counting from 3 to 1, seeing the numbers in your mind's eye. See the number 1 as tall, clear, and bright.

Imagine that you have a mirror to your left. Look into the mirror and see the image of your sadness.

Breathe out. Stretch your index finger up toward the sun.
When it becomes filled with light, bring it down to the mirror.
Use your index finger to cut the image of your sadness in two.

Breathe out. Sweep the two parts of the image out of the
mirror to the left.

Breathe out. Move the mirror to your right. Look into it and
see the image of your life free of sadness. Have all the feelings
that arise with that image.

Breathe out. Open your eyes, cherishing the image and feelings.

Mothers and their babies have always been celebrated in art. I
remember my six-year-old running through the rooms of the Siena
Museum in Italy and returning back to report, "More Madonnas
and Child, Mom!" Mothers with their children are beautiful to
behold; they evoke tenderness, love, home, and all that is best in us.
You are a mother with child. Allow yourself to enjoy the privilege
that confers upon you both a special glow and approval from the
rest of humanity.

RESTRUCTURING

After you've had your baby, your body is still going through major
transitions. What if you aren't feeling beautiful? What if your mind
is filled with depressing thoughts about the way you look? Your body
feels bloated and uncomfortable. You're fearful that you will never
be able to return to your pre-pregnant look. You come out of labor
still carrying most of the weight you gained over the course of nine
months. Can you give yourself a little leeway? Remember the exercise
of intending that you did in chapter 4, *Body cycles* (page 83), in which
you programmed your body to return to its original shape before you
got pregnant. If you let your panicky thoughts take over, you are actually telling your body that it cannot return to the weight and shape

you so fervently desire. Sweep those thoughts off to the left (*Sweep the porch,* page 75) and return to the work of intending your body back into shape. Remember that mind comes before manifestation. Keep your mind steadily on the goal you visualized while doing the *Body cycles* exercise six months ago.

MIRROR OF INTENT
exercise 125

Close your eyes. Breathe out slowly three times, counting from 3 to 1, seeing the numbers in your mind's eye. See the number 1 as tall, clear, and bright.

Looking into a full-length mirror, see your body as it is now.

Breathe out. Sweep that image out of the mirror to the left. See your body going through the stages of losing its roundness until it becomes firm and energetic. Continue looking until you are perfectly satisfied.

Breathe out. Ask to be shown the date at which you will reach your perfect form. See the date—day, month, and year— appearing in the upper right-hand corner of the mirror.

Breathe out. If you are not satisfied with the date, erase it out of the mirror to the left and ask to be shown in the mirror what it is you need to change to reach your goal earlier. It could be your mind, your attitude, or your way of taking care of yourself. See this in images. Address the needs of the images by changing what you need to change.

Breathe out. Look again in the mirror, seeing your perfect form, firm and energetic. See, written on the mirror, the date at which you will reach your goal. Know that you have now set your intent for this to happen in a timely fashion.

Breathe out. Open your eyes, seeing your perfect form with open eyes.

When you are bloated, you need to release the fluids that come with pregnancy, which may take a few days. Next is a little exercise to help with the flushing.

THE VIOLET SQUEEZE
exercise 126

Close your eyes. Breathe out slowly three times, counting from 3 to 1, seeing the numbers in your mind's eye. See the number 1 as tall, clear, and bright.

Imagine that you are standing in a meadow. Look up at the sun, stretch your hands toward the sun, and catch the violet ray from the sun's prism of light.

Breathe out. Surround yourself with the violet ray, from your feet to the top of your head.

Breathe out. Feel the sun pulling the purple ray up. You are caught in a violet spiral that is squeezing and wringing you dry. Keep your feet on the ground while this is happening.

Breathe out. Feel the violet ray dissolving in the light as soon as you have lost the fluids you need to lose.

Breathe out. Open your eyes.

The womb has to shrink in size, and that takes at least six weeks. (Keep the household help for those six weeks so you have time to take care of yourself as well as Baby.) Your abdominal and perineum muscles are extended. To start the process of firming up, you can do Kegel exercises. Following is an exercise that will help, combining physical movement and imagination.

KEGEL IMAGINAL PHYSICAL
exercise 127

Close your eyes. Breathe out slowly three times, counting from 3 to 1, seeing the numbers in your mind's eye. See the number 1 as tall, clear, and bright.

Imagine that you are contracting the sphincter muscles in your perineum, closing the vulva and the anus tightly. What do you sense happening in your thighs, back, and whole body?

Breathe out. Do this physically. Watch what is happening in your body.

Repeat twice more, first imaginally, then physically.

Do this exercise at least five times a day—and any other time you remember to do it. It will firm up all your lower muscles and abdomen.

Only after the first six-week period, and after you have been checked by your doctor or midwife, can you start your restructuring exercises. You can do simple physical exercises like pelvic tilts and modified sit-ups a few days after childbirth, but you must wait six weeks before doing the more strenuous imagery exercises I am about to give you. It is best to have settled into a comfortable rhythm with your baby before starting them.

You are going to practice both of the following exercises three times a day before meals. Remember that when you start menstruating again, you should practice the exercises from the end of one period to the beginning of the next. Stop the exercises during menstruation. If you are breast-feeding and haven't started menstruating again, do the exercises for twenty-one days, stop for seven days, and start again. You can do this for three months in a row if the exercises don't exhaust you.

MOWING THE LAWN
exercise 128

Close your eyes. Breathe out slowly three times, counting from 3 to 1, seeing the numbers in your mind's eye. See the number 1 as tall, clear, and bright.

Imagine that you are mowing an overgrown lawn. All you have is a hand mower. Start mowing the lawn, vertically up and down at first, then horizontally.

Breathe out. As you push the mower, pay attention to your physical sensations: the strain in your legs and arms, your perspiration from the heat. Pay attention to the freshness and smell of the cut grass.

Breathe out. When you are finished mowing, look at your lawn and feel the satisfaction of work well done.

Breathe out. Looking into the mirror of intent, see what you look like now after mowing the lawn, knowing what you intend to look like on the date fixed during *Mirror of intent* (page 226).

Breathe out. Open your eyes.

EYE OF THE NEEDLE
exercise 129

Close your eyes. Breathe out slowly three times, counting from 3 to 1, seeing the numbers in your mind's eye. See the number 1 as tall, clear, and bright.

Sense and see yourself going through the eye of a needle. Have all the physical sensations of squeezing your whole body through the eye of the needle and out the other side. How do you look when you come out on the other side?

Breathe out. Open your eyes, knowing that you are progressing toward being the way you want to be on the date fixed during *Mirror of intent* (page 226).

If you persevere with the restructuring exercises, you will see results. One of my students lost eighty pounds doing just such exercises. But then, as she told me, she was doing them all the time. All the time is too much when you have to take care of your newborn and also resume all your functions as the woman of the house, the mother to your other children (if you have any), and the companion, friend, and lover to your partner.

INTEGRATION

You are now three at home—or more if you have older children. The web of life that was stretched to integrate a new member into your family is closing up again. Hopefully, the fabric of your nuclear community is organizing itself around a new configuration that feels harmonious to all of you. It is good to visualize this web coming together as you bring your family dreamfield into coherence.

MANDALA IN SAND
exercise 130

Close your eyes. Breathe out slowly three times, counting from 3 to 1, seeing the numbers in your mind's eye. See the number 1 as tall, clear, and bright.

You are on the beach with your family. The sand has many different colors. Ask each of the children, starting from the youngest up, to pick a different colored sand. Pick a color for your newborn.

Breathe out. Draw a circle of sand for your newborn, around which each of the other children creates his or her own pattern in a different color.

Breathe out. See that around the central circle, your family's very own mandala begins to appear. When the children are done, you and then your partner finish the mandala to harmonize and create a perfect structure.

Breathe out. See what this mandala looks like; recognize its structure and mood. How do you feel?

Breathe out. Open your eyes, seeing the mandala with open eyes.

Your older child (or children) may find it hard to see himself sup-
planted by an infant in a crib—as he views it. If he is feeling angry that
you are giving Baby all your time, reasoning with him won't help. It is
always best to deal with the situation "through the airways."

THREE FISH
exercise 131

Close your eyes. Breathe out slowly three times, counting from
3 to 1, seeing the numbers in your mind's eye. See the number
1 as tall, clear, and bright.

You are at the beach with your baby and your older child.
Decide to jump into the ocean with both of them. As
soon as you jump into the ocean, see that all three of you
become fish.

Breathe out. See yourselves floating together, letting the
currents move you. Enjoy just moving together in the rhythm
of the ocean.

Breathe out. Hold back while you let your fish-children swim
ahead. See them playing in the coral reefs and among the
colored vegetation of the sea.

Breathe out. Catch up with them and lead them back to shore.

Breathe out. Rise out of the ocean, returning to be yourself
again. Pick up your baby, take the hand of your older child,
and come out of the waters onto the beach. Stretch, lifting
your baby up toward the sun. Have your older child stretch

too. Sing and dance together until the three of you are dry. How does your child respond to Baby now?

Breathe out. Open your eyes.

Your partner has been with you throughout this great adventure, but if you don't integrate him into the all-consuming attention you must give your newborn, he may be having baby blues too. Or, more likely, partner blues. He may be feeling that he has been very patient and attentive and now he needs you to return to him as his friend and lover.

It might be more challenging to find the time and energy, let alone the privacy, to return to being two for an evening. Make that challenge fun and romantic. You can resume your lovemaking two to six weeks after the birth as long as you feel comfortable. If you're exhausted by sleepless nights and your libido is down, which can happen during breast-feeding (frequent breast-feeding suppresses ovulation, thus acting as a form of natural birth control), remember the *Meadow colors* exercise (page 51) you practiced during pre-conception.

THE OTHER HALF OF YOU
exercise 132

Close your eyes. Breathe out slowly three times, counting from 3 to 1, seeing the numbers in your mind's eye. See the number 1 as tall, clear, and bright.

Imagine that you are one half of a circle whose other half is your partner. What do you feel? What is happening?

Breathe out. Open your eyes.

Remember to factor into your new schedule time for the two of you to spend together, free of Baby. You and your partner are the cornerstones of the family you are building together. Without each other, the building collapses. The peace and joy of the family starts with your peace and joy, with each other, together face to face as you started.

Congratulations on having brought your dream into reality. And continue dreaming. Your dreaming is the language that creates. You will be able to create positive outcomes for all the challenges that will inevitably face you with Baby and family by using the tool of your imagination. Don't ever forget to dream!

PART FOUR

Embracing the
Larger Family

8

Fathers and Partners

The dream follows its interpretation.

BABYLONIAN TALMUD, B'RACHOT 56B

OUR MYTHS AND our inner urgings tell us that before becoming separate genders, we were androgynous beings. And it is our longing to be one again that brings us, men and women, back together. It is "we"—not she—that, in uniting through the act of love, will co-create a whole new universe.

Yet many men experience pregnancy as belonging purely in their partner's body, and they resign themselves to being left out of the process. If you are one of those men, think again: you impregnated her, but this doesn't mean that your creative task is over. In fact, it's just beginning. Your task is to continue showering your partner with the warmth of your desire and love so that she may wax fuller and brighter, the precious new life growing in her sustained by your intent and attention. Do not think that you have become superfluous. In fact, your impact is vitally important. You are the life-giving warmth she needs to continue to let creation rise in her like a perfect dream. She needs you.

Your task is to keep your intent and focus on your creation; your mission is to clear away everything that could diminish or weaken or stop that intent from actively enlivening the creation growing within your partner. Like the good farmer, you have planted the seed. Now you must protect, sustain, and nurture what you have planted. Without you, the seed may live but will not fully flourish.

CALLING FORTH

You may have followed your desires only to be surprised and upset when your partner tells you that a baby is on the way. You decide to go along with the pregnancy, belatedly welcoming the idea of becoming a father. Or you see this pregnancy as a biological accident and urge your partner to get rid of it.

If so, think again. From conception onward, the soul of your child is alive and aware. Your child hears and knows what you are planning to do. Many people who have been regressed back into the womb through hypnosis or visualization can attest to this. The worst breakdowns I have witnessed are among men and women who "remember" not being wanted in the womb. Their fear and grief are cataclysmic. They are often surprised by the information and the intensity of their reaction. Many will seek and often get confirmation of the fact by a parent.

Do not leave the conception of your child to chance, even with your beloved partner. It is best to be aware and awake when you decide to conceive. Forging your intent by calling forth your child is the best way to handle such an important event.

TO CALL FORTH A SOUL—FOR FATHER
exercise 133

Close your eyes. Breathe out slowly three times, counting from 3 to 1, seeing the numbers in your mind's eye. See the number 1 as tall, clear, and bright.

Imagine that you are standing in a meadow looking up at the sky on a clear day. See a white cloud floating gently out from the left side of the sky, and see the soul of your child appearing on this cloud.

Breathe out. When your child appears, ask him what you need to do to prepare for his arrival. What changes or preparations must you make for your child to be able to incarnate? Pay special attention to the answer.

Breathe out. When you have heard and seen, promise your child to promptly do what is necessary to secure his arrival. Thank him for being patient.

Breathe out. Open your eyes.

Preparing yourself may mean correcting an emotional imbalance, clearing a mental belief system, or addressing a physical need. It may also be that you need to get your financial situation or your home in order.

You have been in an intimate togetherness with your partner; you have been each other's sole focus. The thought of losing her to another—even if that other is your own child—may be frightening, especially if you were neglected, overlooked, or abandoned by your mother or caretaker in childhood. It is time to take care of that frightened part of yourself or it could hold you back from allowing yourself to grow into greater experience and joy.

WOUNDED CHILD
exercise 134

Close your eyes. Breathe out slowly three times, counting from 3 to 1, seeing the numbers in your mind's eye. See the number 1 as tall, clear, and bright.

See your inner child. Where is he? What is he doing?

Breathe out. Respond to his needs. Find a way to make him happy, contented, and joyfully able to grow.

Breathe out. See your inner child growing perfectly until he is as tall as you are and can look you in the eyes. Then embrace him. As you do, feel that your two breaths become one, that your skins are touching so closely you can't tell the difference between yours and his. What is happening?

Breathe out. Open your eyes.

Taking care of your inner child means that you will never again be neglected, overlooked, or abandoned. This shift from looking for help outside to turning inward and finding your own strength is essential for your future role as a father. After your child is born, you will be faced with new challenges. Becoming your own father to your inner child is an essential step toward preparing yourself to meet those challenges.

Belief systems are harder to discern. They are such familiar ways of thinking that you don't see them unless someone points out to you that you have a mental block. The other way of discerning belief systems is paying attention to the way you repeat yourself in language or patterns of behavior. Most of our mental blocks have to do with how we see ourselves as opposed to how we see others: for example, "I'm the man—I never do the dishes!"

SEE YOURSELF AS OPPOSITES
exercise 135

Close your eyes. Breathe out slowly three times, counting from 3 to 1, seeing the numbers in your mind's eye. See the number 1 as tall, clear, and bright.

See yourself as the victim. Breathe out. See yourself as the perpetrator.

Breathe out. See yourself as the slave; breathe out,
as the master.

Breathe out. See yourself as the old man; breathe out,
as the young man.

Breathe out. See yourself as the pauper; breathe out,
as the king.

Breathe out. Open your eyes.

CONCEIVING CONSCIOUSLY

You are now ready to carry forth your intentions. Before you do, however, think about attuning yourself with your partner. Attunement
means that you and your partner are both of the same mind and heart.
It comes from shared rhythms. You will feel well together if you are
making music together. Your bodies are your unique musical instruments. Start with the simplest of rhythms, your breaths. To perfectly
harmonize your breaths, practice together or separately.

HARMONIZING BREATH
exercise 136

Close your eyes. Breathe out slowly three times, counting from
3 to 1, seeing the numbers in your mind's eye. See the number
1 as tall, clear, and bright.

See yourself in front of your partner. Pay attention to the
rhythm of her breathing. Now watch the rhythm of your own
breathing. What is the difference between these two rhythms?

241

Breathe out. Imagine that a pendulum swings, from left to right and right to left, in the space between you. Feel how the pendulum is finding an in-between rhythm. What happens to your breathing and to the breathing of your partner? How do you feel now?

Breathe out. Open your eyes.

Being attuned is not a fixed state but a constantly changing landscape. Think of it as musical improvisation. The better able you are to improvise counterpoint to the *cantus firmus* or fixed song of your partnership, the better attuned you will be to each other. This is an art that is crucial to your ability to be in a vital relationship. The more you refine your art, the more apt you will be to come to a peak moment of harmonization when you decide to conceive. Being in harmony at the moment of conceiving assures that your child's entrance into this world is at its optimal best.

CONCEPTION

Folk wisdom is clear. It is not good to conceive in anger, fear, sadness, resentment, or against one's will. It is not good to come together while fantasizing about another. In fact, kabbalists believe that the quality of the intent during sexual union has the power to bring "good" to the world. Lack of inward intent or distraction can cause major disruptions in the order and coherence of the universe. Kabbalists and Buddhists alike believe that when two people make love, they create a "spirit body" or love envelope into which form the soul pours itself. Kabbalists call this creating a *diyok'na,* a spirit image that is the garment of the soul. Keeping your love intent strong, clear, and focused on the higher good—on the spirit form to which you both aspire—is crucial. "One is to hallow himself during intercourse so that holy children will descend from him."

The exercise you are about to do is very ancient. It was created by kabbalists to help with conception. Do not read it unless you are ready to sit down and do it. Do it only once.

THE CONCEPTION EXERCISE—FOR FATHER
exercise 137

Close your eyes. Breathe out slowly three times, counting from 3 to 1, seeing the numbers in your mind's eye. See the number 1 as tall, clear, and bright.

Imagine that you are looking up at an emerald-green hill on the summit of which is a magnificent tree. Describe the tree to yourself.

Breathe out. As you start walking up the hill, see your partner walking up on the other side of the hill.

Breathe out. Feel love and the intense desire to meet. As you reach each other, embrace, hold hands, and sit under the tree.

Breathe out. See the blue dome of the sky descending to envelop the tree and both of you.

Breathe out. See a spark of blue light detaching itself from inside the dome, entering the blue space between you and your partner, then speeding into your partner's womb, attaching itself there.

Breathe out. See this bright light in your partner's womb.

Breathe out. The dome of the sky returns to its place in the firmament. The light glows in your partner's womb.

Breathe out. Get up and walk hand in hand down the hill, seeing the glowing light in your partner's womb.

Breathe out. Open your eyes.

You have met imaginally and conceived from the light. Now you must also meet physically. Here is an exercise to enhance your desire and love for each other. You can use it whenever you want to meet physically or simply to stimulate your passion for each other. This is written from the man's point of view: just notice that red is for you and orange for the woman.

MEADOW COLORS—FOR FATHER
exercise 138

Close your eyes. Breathe out slowly three times, counting from 3 to 1, seeing the numbers in your mind's eye. See the number 1 as tall, clear, and bright.

See that you are in a large, very lush green meadow. On the other side of the meadow, see your partner. Feel excited and happy to see her.

Breathe out. As you walk toward each other, see what color she emanates, what color you emanate.

Breathe out. See the colors getting more and more vibrant and warmer. See her becoming more and more brightly orange and yourself brighter and brighter red.

Breathe out. When you come together, see what is created.

Breathe out. Open your eyes, seeing this with open eyes.

You can each practice this exercise as many times as you want. If you know that you are ready to conceive, practice it every night before going to bed. It will stimulate your desire and enhance your love for each other. Remember that focusing on each other to the exclusion of all else except the Mystery that unites you enhances the power of your creation. The greatest power of all is love.

Baby may be conceived immediately, or you may have to wait for his conception. Your time of waiting can seem very long to you. You may be affected by unrequited hopes, or setbacks. Do not despair. Know that waiting is one of the great tools for transformation, used by many religious disciplines to develop inner strength and intent. By gathering your energy, you're building up a great storehouse of power. Use it to help your partner through her disappointment, frustration, and grief when her menses once again appears. Use it to keep faith, to have patience, to be persistent. Use it to come together with ever-mounting love and faith. You are learning courage, the power of the heart to attract to you "a holy soul." When your child finally makes his entry into your lives, he will be the one you were meant to host, the one whom together you called forth with all your heart, with all your soul, and with all your strength.

PREGNANCY

Does your habitually predictable partner have sudden bursts of emotion, unpredictable mood swings, bouts of weeping? Is she being clingy? Is she throwing up in the mornings instead of preparing your breakfast? Are your routines disrupted? While she learns to adapt to the new influx of hormones and the presence of a foreign body (albeit her own child) in her womb, you are presented with a whole new range of challenges and the burning question "Will I be up to the task of handling this?"

Perhaps in the past you could always opt out of a relationship without ruffling too many feathers. But now, with commitment and pregnancy, there's no escaping responsibility. Fears of losing your independence, or your sex life, or exclusivity as your partner's primary concern may be creating a lot of confusion in your mind. Common concerns involved in knowing that Baby is on the way include doubts, worries about the baby's viability or your partner's ability to cope, a sense of unreality about the pregnancy, and detachment from the whole process with accompanying guilt or even resentment. If you are a second- or third (or more)- time dad, because of your partner's exhaustion you may once again have to shoulder all the "female" tasks you most dread. Worse, you will have to reevaluate your ability, both emotionally and financially, to provide for your growing family. Ambivalent, anxious, petrified? Do the following.

THE DARK TRIANGLE
exercise 139

Breathe out, seeing your exhalation as a dark smoke that gathers ahead of you and forms a dark triangle blocking your path. Continue to breathe out the dark smoke, seeing the triangle getting larger as you breathe out. Continue until your breath becomes clearer, then transparent.

Now breathe out strongly against the triangle, breaking it into thousands of pieces.

Breathe out a second time, seeing the pieces dissolving.

Breathe out a third time, seeing that all the wisps of smoke have disappeared and the path ahead is clear.

Open your eyes, seeing the clear path ahead.

The dark triangle works wonders for clearing your mind. If you practice it regularly every morning for twenty-one days, you will have taught your body the habit of automatically clearing your anxiety. You won't have to think about it; the body will know how to let go of anxiety. But if you suffer from chronic crippling anxiety, take a break for three days and then start another round of twenty-one days. Perseverance can make a world of difference.

One way of dealing with anxiety is to squarely face what you need to do to prepare yourself. Making a list of all the things you must take care of may help. This left-brain activity may not be your best solution if you are someone who is overwhelmed by lists, however. Here's a right-brain way of doing it.

MAGICAL BOOTS
exercise 140

Close your eyes. Breathe out slowly three times, counting from 3 to 1, seeing the numbers in your mind's eye. See the number 1 as tall, clear, and bright.

Observing the clear path ahead, put on magical boots, take a huge step forward, and see where the boots have taken you. Whom or what do you encounter?

Breathe out. Open your eyes.

You can always take another step, and another if you need to. The magical boots will show you what your subconscious mind thinks is the most important next step for you to concentrate on now.

CREATING PROSPERITY

It is quite natural for your pocketbook to be one of your first considerations upon hearing about the pregnancy. Even if the pregnancy was planned and joyfully anticipated, it takes a cool man, now that Baby is on the way, to not worry about all the financial ramifications. If your left brain goes into high gear and you start adding up numbers, finish what you're doing. Then switch to your right brain and focus on prosperity. Prosperity always exists in the world of dreaming, and we forget that dreaming can help us manifest it seemingly out of nowhere. Money is a form of energy that creates instantaneous transformation. You give a dollar and get a coffee in return. Can you put your energy out into the world and receive prosperity (in the form of money or otherwise) in exchange? You do it all the time at work. You come up with an *aha!* idea and proceed through all the necessary steps to make your idea manifest.

But with a fixed salary, what can you do? Can you manifest something more? Try it.

PLUCKING PROSPERITY
exercise 141

Close your eyes. Breathe out slowly three times, counting from 3 to 1, seeing the numbers in your mind's eye. See the number 1 as tall, clear, and bright.

Imagine that you lift your hands up toward the sun. Feel your arms elongating, your hands getting closer to the sun, becoming warm and turning into light.

Breathe out. Bring your arms back to their normal length, put your hands of light into your body, gather your best qualities, and, taking your hands out of your body, offer your best qualities to the world.

Breathe out. See what the world is offering back to you. If nothing comes, or something unpleasant does, it means you haven't offered your best qualities.

Breathe out and repeat the motion, putting your hands into your body again, gathering your best qualities and offering them.

Breathe out. Hear the words, "Give and you shall be rewarded tenfold." See what the world is offering back to you. Accept it gratefully.

Breathe out. Open your eyes, seeing with open eyes the gift that has come to you from the world.

If it's hard to believe what you're seeing, suspend disbelief long enough to hold the image in your mind's eye; do that a few times a day. When you are not visualizing your image, let it percolate in the back of your mind. The image will act as a powerful magnet to attract and manifest what you want. To manifest, you must set the date at which that image comes to fruition.

SEEING THE DATE YOUR IMAGES BECOME MANIFEST
exercise 142

Close your eyes. Breathe out slowly three times, counting from 3 to 1, seeing the numbers in your mind's eye. See the number 1 as tall, clear, and bright.

See yourself standing in a meadow. The sky is clear; the sun shines brightly.

Breathe out. Stretch your arm toward the sun. See it getting very long as it reaches toward the sun. Catch a ray of light and draw a circle of light in the upper right-hand corner of the sky.

Breathe out. Now, with a golden pen, write the words "manifest prosperity" around the outer rim of the circle.

Breathe out. Ask to appear in the circle the date (day, month, and year) at which prosperity will manifest for you. Do not force a date; just wait and watch for the first date that appears.

Breathe out. Open your eyes and see this date with open eyes.

You have done everything your right brain requires to set the prosperity process in motion. Remember not to restrict your definition of prosperity to having more financial assets. Prosperity can also mean having a good support system, good friends you can rely on, good community, wholesome food, a warm and loving household. Don't forget to ask for that too. Building belief in the ability of the genie in the bottle (your subconscious right brain) comes from verifying that this strategy works. If you get a result, make a mental note of it and use the same strategy for something else you want to manifest. The more times you verify your results, the more belief you build up.

INABILITY TO CONNECT

Being told you are an expectant father is both exhilarating and, for many men, unreal. You experience your partner's preoccupation with the changes in her body. You're elated and proud but also feel like a stranger in a strange land. This is female territory, a good reason for you to disconnect. Or is it? Like Adam, you are the other half of your Eve. Feeling alienated from her and the pregnancy can have roots in your own inability to balance male and female in yourself. Do you like the male in you? Do you relate to your softer feelings and allow them to manifest?

BALANCE MALE AND FEMALE
exercise 143

Close your eyes. Breathe out slowly three times, counting from 3 to 1, seeing the numbers in your mind's eye. See the number 1 as tall, clear, and bright.

Look into a mirror and see your male side. What do you sense and feel?

Breathe out. Flip the mirror, and in the back mirror see your female side. What do you sense and feel?

Breathe out. See the two mirrors become one common inner space. See your male and female sides turning to face each other. Is the meeting joyful or difficult?

Breathe out. If it's difficult, stretch your hands up toward the sun, fill them with sunlight, bring your hands down into the mirror, and repair what needs to be repaired so that the two sides of yourself, male and female, can meet joyfully.

Breathe out. Open your eyes. See this meeting with open eyes.

COMMUNICATING WITH YOUR PARTNER AND YOUR CHILD

Your child develops in your partner's womb through a nine-month process. Imagine it as the incredibly delicate and exact unfolding of a flower, or as a ballet choreographed by an unknown hand whose every step must be performed perfectly. With your partner's first ultrasound, you will be able to peep into the Garden of Eden where this unfolding takes place. Seeing your child for the first time should make your heart thump! You will feel an intense desire coming over you to protect both mother and child from harm. This will either encourage your sense of responsibility or, perversely, send you into a tailspin of anxiety. You have tools for dealing with anxiety (see *The dark triangle,* page 246). Try those first. But if your fears and needs are too pressing, try not to dump your concerns onto your partner. Instead talk about what makes you fearful or angry or jealous. Or if that stresses her out, learn to do it "through the airways," the dreaming way. Communication is your best strategy!

THE BRIDGE OF LIGHT
exercise 144

Close your eyes. Breathe out slowly three times, counting from 3 to 1, seeing the numbers in your mind's eye. See the number 1 as tall, clear, and bright.

See your partner in front of you. Pay attention to what you feel in your body, describing it to yourself in detail. Where do you feel it? What color is it? What texture?

Breathe out. Take three steps back.

Breathe out. Look at your partner now; what do you feel?

Breathe out. Look into your heart and see the color of your love for her. Send that color as a bridge of light to touch her heart.

Breathe out. Use that bridge to send your words and images to her, making sure that you communicate all you need to communicate at this moment.

Breathe out. Watch to see if anything comes back to you from her.

Breathe out. Open your eyes.

While you might not be able to completely safeguard her peace of mind and happiness, you can be present to her needs. Her greatest need is to have your support. Your child's health depends on your partner's sense of security and self-worth. You are her most important ally, friend, and guardian. If you neglect or abuse her, you are also harming the life unfolding within her. As she watches her child grow perfectly within her, so must you. Half of your child's DNA is yours. He needs to have your loving attentiveness on a consistent basis. As you visualize his perfect unfolding, your little one will respond to your input.

You will need to refer to a chart showing how the fetus develops week by week (the Internet has many examples of pregnancy charts). Each week, check to see what is developing in your baby and visualize him growing perfectly. For example, if the villi (the roots of the placenta) are implanting into the wall of your partner's uterus, see them implanting deeply; if your baby is developing fingers, visualize those fingers growing perfectly.

FATHER GOING INTO THE WOMB TO VISIT HIS CHILD
exercise 145

Close your eyes. Breathe out slowly three times, counting from 3 to 1, seeing the numbers in your mind's eye. See the number 1 as tall, clear, and bright.

Imagine that you are standing behind your partner, your front hugging her back. Have all the sensations of touching her skin with your naked skin. Sense and see becoming one with her for a moment, merging your body and your eyes with her body and eyes.

Turn your eyes inward to travel down to her womb. Your eyes shine like two beams illuminating your way down inside her body to the amniotic sac. When you are there, bring your eyes close to the transparent membrane of the sac and look at your baby floating freely in his clear blue amniotic waters.

Breathe out. Talk to your baby (later on, when your baby has reached the stage of development where his eyes are open, make eye contact with him while talking). Tell your baby all you want to tell him, using words or images. Tell him how much you love him, how much you are looking forward to his arrival.

Breathe out. Tell him of any particular stresses or shocks you may be experiencing. Tell him not to worry, that all is well, that he's safe inside the amniotic sac, tucked under his mother's heart.

Breathe out. Remind your baby of the particular phase of development he's in right now; visualize the perfect development of that part of his body. (Remember, it changes each week, so keep in touch with the weekly changes and visualize them happening perfectly.)

Breathe out. Tell your baby you have to go now but that you'll be back to visit again tonight. Tell him that even though you may be busy with other activities, he's safely in your mind's eye and being taken care of.

Breathe out. Bring your eyes back up to your sockets.

Breathe out. Step out of your partner's body. Feel your front supporting her back. Feel your love for her and for your child enveloping them both.

Breathe out. Step away, knowing that you are continuing to support and love them.

Breathe out. Open your eyes.

Make sure to also talk aloud to your baby. He needs to hear your voice as much as he does his mother's. After birth you will be gratified to see that 80 percent of the time your baby will turn toward your voice rather than that of a stranger. Singing and playing tapping games on his mother's belly are also good ways to relate. Often Baby will respond by kicking back. It is good to stimulate his environment even in the womb. He will react to sounds and stimuli as early as the 16th week.

FATHERS AND ANCESTORS

Visualizing yourself as a support, a tree of life, to your partner and unborn child may have brought to mind that you, too, have a father as well as ancestors whom your child will also share. By giving your child your DNA, you're transmitting your progenitors' and ancestors' patterns. As your partner's belly grows, as you get to peek at your baby on the sonogram screen, your impending paternity will bring back memories of what your dad was like as a father. Do you like the way he was? What if he was an angry, violent, rejecting, or absent father? What if you turn out to be just like your father? In the powerful words of the Bible, God "punishes the children and their children for the sin of the fathers to the third and fourth generation."[23] This statement has always struck me as extraordinarily unfair! But the ancients knew a thing or two about the workings of the subconscious. We cannot dismiss them out of hand.

The very real fear of being "just like Father" can have serious repercussions for your ability to bond with your child. It's time to face that fear now.

REVERSING THE PAST
exercise 146

Close your eyes. Breathe out slowly three times, counting from 3 to 1, seeing the numbers in your mind's eye. See the number 1 as tall, clear, and bright.

Go back to the very first time you ever felt difficulty with your father. See where you are, what is happening, and how old you are.

Breathe out. Imagine that you, the adult, go and stand next to yourself as a child. Tell him you are protecting him now, and he can express what he feels to his father. He must do so in the child's voice.

Breathe out. Tell him that you are going to cut the negative cord between him and his father. Cut the cord. What happens?

Breathe out. Take the child out into a meadow to run and play. Play with him. Tell him he is now free to grow.

Breathe out. See the child beginning to grow through all the stages of childhood, adolescence, and young adulthood until he is the same height as you and you are standing face to face.

Breathe out. Look into the eyes of this other you and embrace him. See and live what happens when you embrace.

Breathe out and open your eyes.

PREPARING FOR LABOR

As the eighth month arrives and you start preparing the nursery and shopping for Baby's arrival, the idea of a child becomes an even stronger reality. By this time, having regularly practiced the exercise *Father going into the womb to visit his child* (page 253), you have imprinted clearly in your mind's eye the image of your child-to-be. In this you are ahead of most dads who, research shows, can only think of their child as an abstract idea or as a five-year-old they're playing rough-and-tumble with. You can actually see your child as the fully formed infant you will soon be holding in your arms.

It is time to start rehearsing the birth with Baby. Think of the planning it takes to prepare for a whitewater rafting trip with your buddies: first, you envision the trip in detail, which helps prepare you for all the eventualities you may encounter and trains you for your forthcoming adventure. This is what sports visualization does. The imaginal script takes the athlete through his performance perfectly. The athlete trains his muscles through his inner seeing. What you are doing—at a distance—is training your baby for his perfect descent into the world.

FATHER REHEARSING THE
BIRTH—THE FLOWER
exercise 147

Close your eyes. Breathe out slowly three times, counting from 3 to 1, seeing the numbers in your mind's eye. See the number 1 as tall, clear, and bright.

Seeing your partner standing in front of you, cross the space between you and merge into her body from behind. See and sense yourself with a big pregnant belly.

Turn your eyes inward into your body. Your eyes are very bright and illuminate the way. Travel down to the amniotic sac.

Breathe out. When you come to the amniotic sac, look in to see your baby floating freely and comfortably in the clear blue amniotic waters.

Breathe out. Make eye contact with your baby, and smile and talk to him, telling him everything you want to say today.

Breathe out. Tell your baby that you and he are going to rehearse his birth. You are going to show your baby exactly what will happen when he is ready to be born. Tell your baby how excited you are at the thought of soon seeing his face and holding him in your arms. You are going to lead your baby through a visualization of his perfect birth.

Breathe out. Visualize your baby turning head down, face toward the sacrum, in the perfect birthing position. See that the cord is floating upward from the belly button, free and unencumbered, and will remain so throughout the birth.

Breathe out. See that your baby's head is resting at the stem of an upside-down flower whose bud is beginning to open up slowly, petal by petal, until the flower is completely open. Breathe out. Now visualize your baby sliding down the stem of the flower in a rush of waters and lubricating oils, the cord floating up freely.

Breathe out. See your baby come out through the wide opening of the flower into a magnificent garden.

Breathe out. See yourself once again outside your partner's body, ready to catch Baby in your hands. Catch him, holding him firmly, as Baby is slippery at birth.

Breathe out. See yourself placing your baby on your partner's chest. Feel the exhilaration and joy as you watch your baby in his mother's arms, as he looks up at your face for the first time. Hear all of nature rejoicing at the coming of your newborn.

Breathe out. Open your eyes.

FACING THE UNKNOWNS OF LABOR

You will know that labor is around the corner when your partner's belly bump is visibly lower. During a preparatory phase called "lightening," the baby has dropped down into your partner's pelvic cavity in preparation for birth. If you and your partner have communicated well with your baby and there are no impediments, he will be in the optimal position for birth, head down at the opening of the cervix and facing backward toward his mother's rear. If your baby is not in the optimal birth position, you can still help by leading your partner through the exercise *Turning baby* (page 147). Do not feel guilty if Baby doesn't turn (it's more difficult when lightening has occurred) or if Baby is not in the optimal position you envisioned. Baby knows best. I had a case where the baby wanted to come feet first. It turned out the umbilical cord was too short; Baby knew enough not to strangle himself. Luckily, today's midwives and doctors are prepared for all eventualities and can deal with them either manually or surgically. This baby's mother practiced the *Drop of oil* (page 127), and Baby came down easily and fast, feet first!

A father-to-be's latent fears surface when the first signs of labor become apparent. This is normal. You would be a cold fish indeed if your emotions weren't stirred up at the thought of what is about to occur! If your mind is a cacophony of questions—Will she be safe? Will Baby have all his toes? Will I be a rock of strength? What if I fall apart?—your best bet is to be well informed. Read through a checklist of all your birth options (chapter 5, page 129) and discuss them with your partner and midwife or doctor. Knowing what to anticipate will give you the calm and courage that may be eluding you just now. Courage comes from *coeur,* a French word meaning heart. Take heart; you will do fine—as do most other men in the labor room.

COURAGE
exercise 148

Close your eyes. Breathe out slowly three times, counting from 3 to 1, seeing the numbers in your mind's eye. See the number 1 as tall, clear, and bright.

See yourself as a lion in a circus. Your trainer is coaxing you to jump through three fire hoops, each one smaller than the preceding one. Have the courage, daring, and determination to jump through the hoops.

Breathe out. As you land on your feet beyond the third hoop, become yourself again. What has changed in you? How do you feel now?

Breathe out. Open your eyes.

If you still feel anticipation and excitement oscillating with fear and the desire to bolt, working with a doula may alleviate your anxieties. After all, she is a pro at this. If you are still feeling queasy about the whole thing and would prefer not to be in on the birth, talk to your partner and the birth professionals helping you. Be honest and upfront about how you feel. They will respect your courage in coming forward.

Stage One of Labor: Dilation and Transition Phases

While you're feeling increasingly vulnerable and anxious about whether you'll be up to the role assigned to you—the supportive, competent partner—your partner may be getting fearful about her first contractions. Most likely she's in false labor, and since you've read up on pregnancy, you can reassure her that these are only the preliminary contractions (called Braxton Hicks) that begin the work of softening her cervix. You will be able to tell because her contractions are not regular, do not get more severe, and will stop if she changes position. Knowing your facts will give you confidence in your ability to deal with what lies ahead.

When your partner's contractions are regular (you will be in charge of timing them) and get progressively more severe, you will know her labor has truly started. If an at-home birth is planned, a phone call to the midwife (and doula if you've hired one) is all you need to think about. If you have planned to have the birth at a hospital or birth facility, your major concern will be getting your partner there. Don't rush there until either the doctor or your partner tells you it is time. When your partner stumbles around as if she's drunk and tells you she can't see straight, it's definitely time. You have obviously thought ahead about how to transport yourselves to your chosen facility. All you need to do now is implement your plan. Don't get panicky if your well-laid plans get messed up. Trust the dreaming; it has a way of smoothing out the most thorny difficulties, including traffic jams.

BLUE PATHWAY—FOR FATHER
exercise 149

Breathe out all that tires you, obscures you, upsets you as a dark smoke that floats out the window and is absorbed by the vegetation outside.

Breathe in the blue-gold light from the sky. See it entering your nostrils, filling your throat and your mouth.

Breathe the blue-gold light slowly out of your mouth, creating a path of blue-gold light all the way from your home to the hospital. See the blue-gold light arriving at the hospital and, as the door opens, entering and filling the corridor all the way into the birthing room.

Breathe out. See the two of you in the car, following this path of light to the hospital, knowing that it will open up the way to your destination. See the two of you arriving safely and being welcomed into the sunlit birthing room where your partner will continue to labor peacefully in the light.

Breathe out. Open your eyes.

If you're usually the one calling the shots, here's where your role switches to that of facilitator. Your partner's needs come first! At the hospital, your role will be threefold: keeping her safe from interruptions; interfacing with the doctor, midwife, and nurses; and making decisions for her when she cannot do so herself. For some men, labor may be their first on-the-spot training for fatherhood: learning to forget themselves in caring for another. But since you've practiced the exercises, you're way ahead of the game. You've been in your partner's body and helped her carry. You'll be able to sense and anticipate her every need, whether she wants a back rub, a foot massage, or for you to hold her hand. And if she doesn't want you near her at this moment, that's all right too. She's in the lead!

You're the timekeeper. Her contractions are getting stronger, helping open up the cervix through which your baby must pass. When you see a contraction starting, sound the breath *beuu* with her. Make it very soft.

BEUU BREATHING—FOR FATHER
exercise 150

Breathe out slowly as if through a long straw that is starting
way down in your lower abdomen. Breathe out on the sound
of "beuu." At first you make this sound in your mouth, then
slowly bring it down into your throat. Eventually it should
sound like the wind rustling through the leaves of a tree. Try
to make the sound very smooth; imagine it as a long, smooth
ribbon of light. Practice this breathing until it feels effortless
and nearly silent.

By modeling the breath for her, you are supporting her in breathing
out slowly and smoothly through each contraction.

If dilation isn't progressing (which your birth practitioner will
determine), use the sound *deee,* which will help her cervix to dilate.

DEMETER, DOORWAY OF THE
MYSTERIOUS FEMININE—FOR FATHER
exercise 151

Breathe out on the sound *de.* Keep the sound high, *deeee . . . ,*
holding the sound as long as is comfortable and visualizing
your partner's lower parts opening from the inside out. See her
cervix opening up.

Breathe in. Visualize the breath in as golden light that flows
down to her cervix, coating it with warm, golden sunlight.

Repeat three times.

Breathe out. Open your eyes.

Talking her through the exercises in a soft, low voice (in her left ear is best; it will speak straight to her right brain and subconscious) will help tremendously. Practice this next exercise on yourself to verify its efficacy.

DROP OF OIL—FOR FATHER
exercise 152

Close your eyes. Breathe out slowly three times, counting from 3 to 1, seeing the numbers in your mind's eye. See the number 1 as tall, clear, and bright.

Imagine catching a ray of sunlight in a small crystal vial. Hold the vial a moment in your hands. See the sunlight in the vial becoming a liquid golden oil.

Breathe out. Drink the oil, seeing it going down into your hips and your pelvic bone structure. See it coating your whole bone structure, then moving into your muscular structure.

Breathe out. See how the sunlit oil begins to expand into all of your pelvic area. See the muscles becoming soft and pliant, the bone structure opening up and breathing with the sunlit oil. See the pelvic floor softening and opening up.

Breathe out. See the drop of oil flowing down into your anus and continuing to expand and soften your tissues.

Breathe out. Open your eyes.

If you are coaching your partner, replace the last two sentences with the following:

Breathe out. See the drop of oil flowing down into your womb and continuing to expand and soften your tissues. See your cervix opening easily. See the skin of your perineum—supple, golden, and elastic—stretching easily.

Breathe out. Imagine your baby rotating into the right position and, coated in oil, slipping out easily.

Breathe out. Open your eyes.

In between contractions, remind her to rest. And don't forget to rest too!

Don't tell her to open her eyes. This is her dreaming time. As long as she is in the dream state, she won't feel pain as pain, but as pressure. It is only when she is disturbed that pain flares up. Your job is to protect her from disturbances and unnecessary interruptions. And if she is interrupted, which will inevitably happen, help her get back into the dreaming state by becoming very quiet yourself.

The most intense part of her labor is the transitional phase, which lasts no longer than fifteen minutes to one hour. The contractions are close together, and peaks are long. This is the phase in which you will want to talk her through *Riding the wave (2)* (page 176), which I have repeated here for your convenience.

As the contraction begins, blow out dark smoke and with it any pain, tension, or fear you have. See the smoke being absorbed by the vegetation outside.

Inhale the blue-gold light from the sky, seeing it flow warm and comforting into your body—melting, softening, widening everything it touches.

Sense and see it melting, softening, widening your forehead; melting, softening, widening your jaw; melting, softening, widening your shoulders . . . chest . . . abdomen. See the light spreading out, flowing into your womb, coating your womb with melting, softening, warm golden light. See the warm golden light surrounding the head of your baby, melting the cervix, melting the vaginal muscles, the perineum, inner thighs, calves, feet.

Breathe out and return to your natural breathing, feeling the pause after the surge and knowing that all is well and in order.

Lengthen the pronunciation of the words "melting," "softening," and "widening." This will help her ride the wave of sensations that comes with each new contraction. Do this imagery with her or, if she's too engaged to hear you, for her. Support her lower back with your hands. She'll feel the warmth and love your hands are communicating.

As her cervix reaches full dilation, she will begin to show signs of exhaustion. If she cries out that she can't take this anymore, that she wants an epidural *now,* which the doctor can't give her at this point, remind her that feeling overwhelmed is typical of the short transition phase she's in just now. Tell her it'll soon be over and she'll be entering the second stage of labor, where contractions are interspaced with long pauses. Remind her that she'll soon be in a proactive role pushing her baby out.

Stage Two: Pushing and Delivery

Suddenly the raging storm of furiously paced contractions is over. You will both be surprised by the quiet that follows. Your partner now has time to rest between her longer-spaced contractions. You can remind her to practice *Ocean of light (2)* (page 149), *In the hand of the Divine* (page 149), or *White cloud* (page 177) exercises to help her with resting and recouping her energy. On the rise of a contraction, encourage her to push. Do not allow anyone to tell her to push when she's not having a contraction.

While your partner is enjoying a well-deserved change of pace, you can position yourself behind her to support her back. Or you can help hold her while she squats. If you're in a hospital, you'll be asked to step back as nurses take over and the doctor is called in. They will be telling her when to push and how to push. If you can get a word in, remind her of the *Beuu* exercise and *Drop of oil*. Tell her to sound out the *beuu* LOUDLY and to push with all she's got, just as she would to push out a hard stool. *Drop of oil* will help. You'll be pushing with her (and so will everyone else in the room); you won't be able to help yourself, and that will give her the extra oomph! she needs to push the baby out.

Soon the doctor will call you to the foot of the bed to witness the "crowning": the moment when your baby's hairy (or bald) little head first appears at the mouth of the vagina. Get ready to catch your little one when he comes out. Remember that he'll be quite slippery because he's covered with vernix, a thick white cream that has protected his skin in the amniotic waters. So hold him firmly but without squishing him. Think of a squirming fish you've just pulled out of the water.

Now place your newborn on your partner's chest. And rejoice!

You have all come through this safely. This is your and your partner's "crowning" achievement. At long last, you get to meet the unique little being you have created together. Don't worry about Baby's first cry. It may or may not happen. With DreamBirth babies, more often than not, the first breath is quiet and easy. The baby will open clear eyes to this new world and will calmly search for his mother's face and yours, as soon as he hears your voices.

We leave you to this joy, as nothing must interrupt this perfect moment of communion.

BONDING

Is it not a quasi-universal belief that mothers are more nurturing than fathers? Well, think again! Researcher Ross Parke has long established that males can be just as caring and involved as females. If given free rein, fathers will hold, rock, coo, and cuddle their newborns just as much as their partners will. We all know how mesmerizing an infant is. We can't stop looking! This phenomenon is called "engrossment." Fathers are just as engrossed as mothers are.

Your bonding starts at birth with seeing and holding your baby. Physical closeness is important and will sweep away any kind of exhaustion you might be feeling because of what your partner and you have just been through. Once you hold that little one close, love will sweep all other emotions away. And if the bonding doesn't occur right away, don't worry. It will happen in time. Here is your basic bonding exercise.

BONDING WITH YOUR
NEWBORN—FOR FATHER
exercise 153

Breathe out a light smoke and with it all that disturbs you, pains you, or obscures you. With the inhalation, breathe in the blue-gold light from the sun.

See and feel this light entering into your nostrils, flowing down into your throat.

See it as a great river of light flowing down your back, into your legs, feet, toes. See it emanating from your toes as long blue-gold antennas of light.

Now see this river of light traveling up your legs into your pelvis and to your heart, which becomes a great, glowing blue light.

Breathe out. From the light in your heart, cast a blue-gold net over your baby. Feel and see your baby bathed in the warmth of this protective light and send your love through each strand of light. See and feel how your baby responds.

Breathe out. See the light flowing up to your shoulders and into your arms, hands, and fingers, stretching out of your fingers like long antennae of light. Hold your baby in the crook of your left elbow, near your glowing heart. See and feel how your baby is being bathed in love and soothing blue-gold light. Feel this connection in all of your body, mind, heart, and soul.

Breathe out. Open your eyes, seeing the connection to your baby with open eyes.

When you have to be away from your baby, imagine the blue-gold mesh stretching all the way from your heart to him. While physically separated from you, your baby will continue to experience your comforting presence and feel safe. If you are interested in exploring more, you will find additional bonding exercises starting on page 196.

Once a father, always a father! As your newborn grows, he will elicit in you your most tender thoughts and fondest hopes. If you continue practicing your bonding exercises, this response can only grow. However difficult the challenges ahead, never stop dreaming for your child and with him. Never stop communicating. You will find that fatherhood turns out to be a uniquely precious and fulfilling adventure.

When Your Child Dreams You

*Dreams pass into the reality of action. From the actions stems the dream
again; and this interdependence produces the highest form of living.*

ANAÏS NIN

WITH HER TEN fingers and ten toes, your little one wiggles the
mystery of creation at you. She is the awesome and wondrous embodiment of your dreaming. The power of her presence is beyond your
wildest hopes. She is your dream made flesh, clothed in warm skin,
plump folds, eyes tantalizingly familiar and unfathomable—and she
is a revelation!

Her reality is more tangible than your dreaming could ever prepare
you for. She bursts forth with a life of her own, like a subterranean
river surging out of the ground where you least expect it, forging a
way of its own making. You may think that you were just the hollow
receptacle to the flow of life. But, no, you each gave your baby parts
of yourselves. Yet beyond the two of you, her reality, as she emerges
from the birth canal, is palpable. And the journey of discovering who
she is begins.

You step into the unknown. Your little one is beginning to reveal
"the land that (she) will show you," but she won't let you see beyond
her needs, her milky smell, her fuzzy skin, her cooing and giggles, her

gentle snores. Be patient and surrender to her magic. She will show you the way, step by step, day by day.

You thought you were the creator. Your child—your dream come true—is now creating you, the new you that you never dreamed you could become. How will you respond to her molding of you?

If all has gone well, your first experience of her is one of undiluted joy, amazement, and ravishment. Her arrival triggers a peak experience, one of very few in a lifetime. Time slows to a shimmering quietness and every gesture, every glance, every smile hovers at the edge of perfection. In the very first instant of her presence, she has toppled you into the mystery of life. You have touched the creative source and been renewed.

But while this ravishment may long continue to inform the deeper layers of your being, reality will soon reassert itself and you will be plunged back into the daily round of preoccupations. This doesn't mean you don't love your baby as completely as in those first moments, but right now you must master the art of diapering a slithering infant or soothing her frantic cries. Will she latch on? Will she gain weight? Why does she cry? Have you done something wrong?

In the throes of joy, sadness creeps in and maybe even guilt, resentment, and fear. Why the guilt, resentment, and fear? Experiencing is not just black or white. Your baby will lead you a merry dance of up and down, wet and cold, milk and poop. Ravished by joy and exhaustion, flooded with sensations that are unrelenting and inescapable, you will be driven to feel acutely the hell of your paradise. Rashes, regurgitations, diarrheas, fevers hound your sleepless nights. Welcome to the joys of parenthood.

What if your little one is not what you expected? What if she has Grandpa's big ears or Mom's black mole? What if . . . What if your joy is shattered by anxiety for her health or horror at her disabilities? What if your little one doesn't make it through the birth canal alive or leaves soon after birth? In all instances, remember that she is a gift given to you, her parents, for an allotted time only. She will grow up and walk away into her life. "He is all mine!" said a friend at her son's birth. "Thank heaven you have twenty years to work on this" was my answer.

While you thought you were riding your dreaming, the dreaming in fact now rides you. Or should we say there is a dialogue? Like a surfer, you will learn to surrender to the wave, but don't forget to surf it with

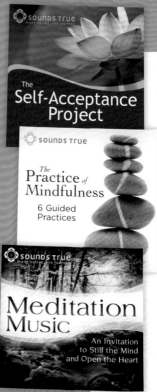
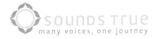

all the mastery dreaming has taught you. And always remember that she, the precious manifestation of your dreaming, is never yours to possess.

OCEAN OF LIGHT (3)
exercise 154

Close your eyes. Breathe out slowly three times, counting from 3 to 1, seeing the numbers in your mind's eye. See the number 1 as tall, clear, and bright.

See, feel, and remember that like all human beings, you and your baby are part of the great flow of life.

Breathe out. See the great flow of life as an ocean of light that picks you and Baby up and gently brings you to the top of a wave.

Breathe out. Sense and see how you and Baby are turning into light, every cell in your bodies becoming light. See that you both become one with the ocean of light.

Breathe out. Ride the wave of light as it rolls onto the beach.

Breathe out. Now return to be yourself, holding Baby in your arms. Sit and contemplate the rolling waves on the ocean of light. Listen to the roar of the waves and the soft breathing of your baby.

Breathe out. Give thanks and rejoice at the weight and scent of Baby as she lies trustingly in your arms, her head close to your heart.

Breathe out. Open your eyes.

Baby comes with a big question mark and a tough lesson. As parents—for that is what you have become, for better and for worse—you are being taught to love what you have and to find what is lovable in her. Love her with her big ears, her quirks, and her vulnerability. Love her and be grateful. She comes and goes at the will of the dreaming that you are learning to serve and trust.

Be grateful every moment of every day and night, through joy, through fear, through wonder, through disgust. You are being fine-tuned to forget yourselves for another. You are the lucky ones, destined to reach that hidden point of no duality, that unconditional love that only a parent can have for his or her child (natural or adopted).

As she leads you through the relationship dance and you respond, never give up on the give-and-take of dreaming together. Continue to see the dream that she is, and then dream her some more. Is she a nightmare, a repetitive dream, a busy or clear dream? At different times, she'll be each one of those. Respond to the necessity of her dreaming with pure intent, and you will reach a presence of intimacy with your baby that verges upon mystery. Cherish it and guard it well. There is nothing like dreaming the great dream of parenthood!

THE PARADOX OF PEACE
exercise 155

Close your eyes. Breathe out slowly three times, counting from 3 to 1, seeing the numbers in your mind's eye. See the number 1 as tall, clear, and bright.

Imagine joy and pain as two dream objects. Note in which hand you hold joy, in which hand pain.

Breathe out. Bring both hands, with their dream objects, palm to palm. Feel the heat and moisture.

Breathe out. When your two hands are so connected that they feel like one, open your hands like a cup. What do you have now in your hands?

Breathe out. Open your eyes, seeing this with open eyes.

The image that has emerged in your cupped hands is paradox, the state of peace beyond duality that the prophet Isaiah speaks about. "The wolf also shall dwell with the lamb, and the leopard shall lie down with the kid; and the calf and the young lion and the fatling together; and a little child shall lead them."[24] Whatever your image is of peace, let it shine in you. Keep visualizing it. Let it guide you through the challenges of parenthood. Remember, "a little child shall lead" you, the child of your dreaming that has brought you the magical presence of your child!

EXCERPTS OF DREAMBIRTH STORIES
BY CLAUDIA ROSENHOUSE-RAIKEN

EFFECTS OF THE "GARDEN" EXERCISE

Desiree was in triage. She was expecting a second child, and her water had already broken. Second births tend to be quick, and the room was in chaos: people rushed in and out, her husband was not there, machines buzzed, and everyone felt the pressure of time. I wasn't accustomed to so much confusion and realized something was missing. "Have I taught you the garden?" I asked. Within minutes, not only Desiree but also the climate of the entire room switched, completely calming down. A half hour later, her daughter was born in an easeful and calm atmosphere, which was gratefully acknowledged by the nurses and doctor!

Verification of *The garden—to prepare for an operation* came from Cynthia, a doula who had studied DreamBirth with the initial group; she had been an OB/GYN nurse for several years in the same hospital and knew the doctors well. Cynthia finally overcame some skepticism and used *The garden—to prepare for an operation* with a birthing mom. She called me, exulting: "I can't believe it! It really works! The atmosphere was so different!"

BACK LABOR AND WRAPPED CORD

Since using DreamBirth, I have observed in my clients an almost nonexistent rate of back labor and lower incidence of cord wrap. *Rehearsing the birth—the flower* alone is responsible for the remarkably small number of back labor problems. Out of two hundred births only one was a back labor, and only for part of the time (in the United States the normal incidence of back labor is about 30 percent). *Rehearsing the birth—the flower* is also responsible for a decrease in cord wrap.

A client who had moved back to Chile called me long distance, in obvious distress. She was pregnant with her second child, due in a few weeks, and the ultrasound had shown that the cord was wrapped several times not only around the neck, but also around the left leg. I had her do the DreamBirth exercise to untangle the cord and reminded her of the exercise we used to rehearse the birth. She asked if she should keep untangling the cord. Experience has proved that the imagery can work right away, so I encouraged her to "practice the birth" and only untangle the cord if she had trouble seeing it "freely floating" in the exercise.

Two weeks later she emailed me that her most current ultrasound had shown the cord to be freely floating. She had an easy, uneventful birth very shortly afterward.

BABY'S DESCENT

One of my clients, Annette, who had taken an epidural, was opening and effacing very nicely, but the baby was very high and seemed to be staying there. On one of my trips to get my client ice chips, I bumped into the doctor coming out of another birthing room. Privately she confided, "You'll see—she'll [my client] be a C-section. That baby is too high up. It'll never come down."

I returned with the ice chips and said to both the mother and her husband, "Let's concentrate on seeing the baby sliding down the stem (part of our *Mother rehearsing the birth—the flower)*, coming out, and being put on your chest." In less than an hour the baby descended from -2 station to +1 station and my birthing mom successfully pushed the baby out. We were all pleased, no one more so than the doctor. This experience has repeated itself twice with that same doctor. Even though the doctor communicated concern to the patients or sometimes just to me, the babies descended in the way just described.

TWEAKING THE BABY'S POSITION DURING TRANSITION

My client Ty illustrates a rather dramatic example of tweaking the baby's position during the transition phase of labor.

When we got to the hospital, she was 8 centimeters and still very relaxed during her contractions. Given her composure, it was a surprise to the doctor and nurses that she was already in the transition phase. Many weeks before her labor started, Ty had told me she was planning to take an epidural when she reached 8 centimeters, and although she seemed to be dealing quite beautifully, she did not change her mind. She asked for the epidural as soon as she was checked and was told she was completely effaced and 8 centimeters open. She progressed very nicely to 9.5 centimeters with the epidural, and then the progress stopped.

After almost two hours, the doctor came in and examined her. The doctor's estimation was that the baby had twisted a little. "When this happens the baby's head is not pressing in the right way," the doctor explained. "We'll see if you can open fully. If you don't after another hour or two, I'm afraid we might have to consider a C-section."

After the doctor left, I had Ty imaginally bring her eyes down to the baby and check its position. Inner sight is uncannily accurate. Ty reported that the baby had turned slightly to the left. I asked her to imaginally transform her arms and hands into light, go in to where the baby was, and help get it into the perfect position. She told me that she was centering the baby's head to her own pubic joint. I asked her if the baby stayed in the right position when she took her hands off. She said yes.

For the next fifteen to twenty minutes, I had her check imaginally. Every time, the baby was correctly positioned, but even more exciting was that all the signs of being completely open and ready to push were there. The doctor arrived, exclaiming that she had never witnessed a baby turning at that point in the labor, especially with an epidural: "This is fantastic!" Thirty-five minutes later Ty's daughter was born.

REVERSING FUNNELING, STOPPING EARLY LABOR

Denise was not at all sure what she thought about imagery. She was willing to practice the exercises but was quite skeptical that anything would come of it. About week 23 she called in tears. She had spent the previous evening at the hospital with early contractions. Although the contractions had stopped, the ultrasound showed that her cervix had thinned and that it was starting to open toward the side of the amniotic bag (not toward the side of the vaginal canal). This condition is called "funneling." The only answer, according to her doctor, was bed rest for the remainder of her pregnancy to make sure the cervix did not continue to thin and open.

Denise was convinced this meant the end of her pregnancy. I taught her the exercise called *Tying the pouch* to stop premature contractions. Two weeks later at her next exam, Denise was told that her cervix had reversed direction and had thickened. The funneling, however, was still there.

At our next visit Denise reported her progress and told me she had changed the exercise slightly. She was visualizing a pouch now with two sets of ties, an inner one and an outer one. Excited at the results, she often practiced her new and improved exercise. Two weeks later the ultrasound showed that the funneling was gone and she was off bed rest!

The doctor said she had never, ever seen funneling reverse itself, or read about it, or heard about it!

. . . AND RESTORES A BABY'S HEART RATE

Rosanna's cervix had started to open quite early. To ensure a safe delivery she was put on bed rest, and her baby's lungs were helped to mature. At week 32, Rosanna's cervix was open 3 centimeters. Although she did *Tying the pouch* daily, Rosanna, a very cautious person, decided to stay on bed rest even though the opening had stabilized. The plan was that at 36 weeks she would get off bed rest and start to move and lead a normal life. We all expected that once her labor started, it would go quickly.

When her contractions started, Rosanna, accompanied by her husband, started walking around the hospital hallways to help stimulate her labor. As is normal during prodromal labor, the contractions were erratic and started to slow down. Because her water had broken, the doctor decided to help the labor along by giving her Pitocin.

When Rosanna realized that she had to stay in bed (or close by) so they could closely monitor the baby, and that she could no longer walk around, her mood switched. She felt confined and angry and became silent and sullen. Her dream of an easy, natural birth was gone. The Pitocin drip had barely started and the contractions were quite mild, but the baby's heart rate started to dip after every contraction. This was not a good sign. If the baby was doing this at such an early stage, she would never be able to tolerate labor; a potentially easy labor might turn into a C-section. I asked Rosanna to go inside and connect with her baby. "I can't see her face," she said quite petulantly. "Rosanna," I persisted, "your eyes in imagery can travel. Connect with your baby. Look at her face and eyes."

Perhaps because her husband could also feel the sullen, simmering anger, he put on some Russian pop music (Rosanna and her husband are Russian). As Rosanna closed her eyes, she imagined picking her baby up and dancing with her. She saw the baby smiling. When Rosanna opened her eyes, the mood had lifted. I looked at the monitor: no more dips! The baby's heart rate, from that moment on, stayed reassuringly perfect, exactly the way the nurse and doctor wanted the baby to react to the contractions. Rosanna's daughter was born five hours later.

INCREASING BABY'S RATE OF GROWTH

Karen was upset that one of her twin babies was quite a bit smaller than the other. She knew this was normal but wanted to use imagery to help them grow equally and to a healthy but manageable size. She used *Tying the pouch* to make sure her cervix stayed long, which it did. She reached full term without going on bed rest, an unusual occurrence for twins in the United States.

Karen used a very simple exercise each time she ate. Her diet already consisted of food with very high nutritional value; she wanted only the best for both herself and her babies. During every meal she would visualize the broken-down food becoming a flow of light, going equally to each of her children. The exercise worked; at birth they were of almost equal weight.

LIZ'S BIRTH

Liz's water broke, and her labor came on suddenly and furiously, untypical for a first birth. The sudden start of the contractions and the intensity of her pain made Liz forget all that she had practiced.

All Liz wanted, expressed through her tears and panicked eyes, was an epidural. That changed, however, as she began to do *Drop of oil for releasing contractions,* where you breathe in light that melts and softens each part of the body that needs to stay relaxed—the forehead, jaw, shoulders, and so on. Because it seemed to calm her, I kept walking her through the imagery. *The garden—to prepare for procedures* exercise must have been fully operational that night because a normally quite conservative hospital (in Long Island, New York) allowed her to birth upright while following the images. After thirty minutes of continually repeating the words of the exercise to her, I figured she (and I) might need some silence. Wrong. She looked at me, panic-stricken. All she could say was, "Words, words. Do the words."

DREAMBIRTH FACILITATES CONNECTION
BETWEEN UNBORN CHILD AND MOTHER

DreamBirth's greatest gift is the connection it engenders between the unborn child and the mother and father. Practicing *Going into the womb to visit your child* daily allows the connection to be experienced viscerally. Perhaps the best way to illustrate this is by quoting one of my clients, Sharon, who wrote about her experience during labor:

> While I was in labor, I felt very close to my baby—like we were going through it together—and I could imagine and "see" her safe and okay in there, even though it was a painful experience for me . . . I never once felt like giving up or panicked when that stupid fetal heart rate monitor slipped out of position or the batteries died, because I truly felt calm and that the baby was just fine.

After witnessing many similar experiences, I can confidently claim that Sharon's experience echoes that of probably every mother who has used DreamBirth. The imagery establishes a strong, healthy, easeful, and positive connection between Mother and Baby from the very beginning—sometimes even from before conception—so that the bonds at birth are as tremendously beautiful and tender as they ought to be.

ACKNOWLEDGMENTS

I WANT TO thank the seven remarkable women who accompanied me throughout this journey: Mia Hadjes, Judith Hallett, Ruth Lawyer, Claudia Raiken, Jackie Schiff, Izetta Stern, and Cynthia Zinser. Without them, *DreamBirth* would never have seen the light of day. These dedicated birth professionals shared their expertise with me and voiced their clients' needs, which inspired me to write some eight hundred imagery exercises to help with all manner of issues concerning conception, pregnancy, labor, and bonding. The most potent 160 of these exercises for the reader are featured in this book. Thank you for your support and belief in the work. Thank you for so faithfully turning up for seven years to our Wednesday sessions, for your critical input, for testing the exercises, and for taking DreamBirth to the many moms- and dads-to-be.

Two other powerful women dropped in on our DreamBirth classes and contributed their expertise: Elizabeth Poole, a specialist in neonatal craniosacral work with mothers and infants, and Dr. Bonnie Buckner, who got us a grant for a clinical study of DreamBirth's efficiency in helping mothers through labor (as of now, we are still searching for a hospital that would be open to such a study).

I also want to thank all the moms and dads who practiced the exercises, trusted in the process, and gave their feedback. It was invaluable in refining the exercises' efficacy as well as when it came time for me to choose which ones to incorporate in this book.

Thanks also to the godmother of my book, Gay Walley. Gay was my first reader, an enthusiastic supporter, and a critical voice all along the way. I also feel enormous gratitude to my dear friend and agent Jane Lahr, who encouraged me throughout the process and gently goaded me to get the book finished. My first editor, Joanne Zazzaro, coached me through the initial round of editing and through English punctuation—not my strong suit.

My publisher, Nancy Smith, was immediately onboard, which gave me a huge boost in getting the book ready. As for my editor, Haven Iverson, I am most grateful for her acute and valuable comments and her reminder to me to give my *wow* best to the process.

O'Mara Leary, administrator of the School of Images (SOI, my nonprofit organization to disseminate the use of imagery throughout the world), is a constant supporter and a standup comic to boot. If I needed a break, I was sure to get a refreshing quip from her and a friendly reminder that I would get through this. She was an invaluable help in editing the material for the DreamBirth tapes.

Students coming in and out of classes at SOI were supportive of the process and eager to hear news of the book's progress.

SOI's housekeeper, Marlita Pereira, deserves a special mention. She is the mother in our community. She takes care of all our needs and protects me from what she sees as possible intrusions to my writing. I thank you, Marlita, for pouring your loving attention on all of us and showing us in action what a truly loving mother is.

A special mention goes to my friend Patricia Masters, who died young, leaving two small children. She urged me to write this book and during our last conversation three weeks before she died, shared some deep thoughts about the soul connection between parents and their children.

Being a mother has been the most transformative experience of my life. As I spent days and nights writing, my son, Sam, remained an amused and enthusiastic supporter. Many of the exercises have been inspired by our relationship. I learned so much from him—not only through our daily encounters but also in the dreams I had about him, and in the dreams he shared with me. My fondest wish is for all my readers to learn and grow from dreaming with their child.

For Surgical Procedures and Medical Tests

DO THIS EXERCISE whenever you are about to have a medical procedure or surgery. The baby is included in this version, but when you aren't pregnant, or if you are sharing it with a family member or friend who is about to undergo surgery, omit the parts about the baby. After thirty-five years of teaching this exercise, I can safely say that it will transform your experience and that of your doctors, shorten the time the operation takes, and hasten your recovery.

THE GARDEN—TO PREPARE FOR PROCEDURES
exercise 156

Close your eyes. Breathe out slowly three times, counting from 3 to 1, seeing the numbers in your mind's eye. See the number 1 as tall, clear, and bright.

You are walking around the base of a circular wall. Above the wall, you see the tops of trees. Walk until you find the gate. The key is in the lock. Open the gate and walk into the garden.

Breathe out. What does your garden look like?

Breathe out. Walk deeper into the garden and find a patch of thick, soft, emerald-green grass next to a tree and a running brook.

Breathe out. Lie on the grass in the shade of the tree and listen to the sounds of the brook and the birds, feeling how your body rhythms become attuned to the rhythms of nature.

Breathe out. Now invite those you trust to come into the garden one by one and sit in a semicircle around your head. Feel their love and attentiveness to you and your unborn child.

Breathe out. When all of your witnesses have come in and sat down around you, and you feel comfortable and at ease, *show your body in a precise visualization exactly what is going to happen and ask permission of your body to allow the procedure* your doctor is about to perform.

Breathe out. If your body refuses permission, ask your body what it needs in order to accept the procedure. Respond to the needs of your body in images.

Breathe out. Once your body has given permission, ask permission of your baby to allow the procedure.

Breathe out. If your baby refuses permission, ask your baby what he needs in order to accept the procedure. Respond to the needs of your baby in images.

Breathe out. Invite your doctor, assistants, and nurses to come into the garden with their medications and tools. When they stand before you, see how the sunlight pours down onto their heads and into their arms and hands so that everything they touch—medications, tools, your body—turns into light.

Breathe out. See that all is done perfectly. Check with your baby that all is well.

Breathe out. See the doctor, assistants, and nurses leaving.

Breathe out. Feel all of your loved ones still around you, guarding and protecting you and your baby; feel their love and their joy. When you are ready, see them go one by one out of the garden. The gate closes after the last one, and you are alone with your baby.

Breathe out. Feel the rhythms of nature; feel your body and your baby breathing with the rhythms of nature.

Breathe out. When you are ready, get up and slowly walk out of your garden with your baby tucked safely under your heart (or held in your arms), close the gate, and take the key or put it in a place where you will always be able to find it.

Breathe out. Walk into your future confident and serene.

After every surgical procedure, or simply to clear out toxins from anesthesia or medications, do this next exercise (also presented earlier in the book).

THE RIVER RUNS THROUGH
exercise 157

Close your eyes. Breathe out slowly three times, counting from 3 to 1, seeing the numbers in your mind's eye. See the number 1 as tall, clear, and bright.

Imagine that you are in your garden or in a meadow. You are lying on the thick, soft emerald-green grass. Listen to the sound of a stream nearby. Get up and go look at the stream. The water is very clear and you can see the sandy bottom.

Breathe out. Take off your clothes and lie down in the stream with your head toward the source of the stream. Feel the water flowing from head to feet all around you, cleaning and clearing you, opening up the pores of your skin.

Breathe out. Now see and feel the stream entering the pores of your skin, flowing through your body and out the soles of your feet, washing out all the toxins from your body until your body becomes as translucent and clear as the stream.

Breathe out. Rise out of the water and stretch yourself in the sunlight until you are dry. Returning to your clothes, see that your old clothes are gone. New, clean, white clothes, loose and soft, are awaiting you. Put them on and feel clean and refreshed.

Breathe out. Open your eyes, seeing this with open eyes.

Do the following exercise when you have had a tear or an incision from a surgical procedure, such as a C-section.

WOUND REPAIR (2)
exercise 158

Close your eyes. Breathe out slowly three times, counting from 3 to 1, seeing the numbers in your mind's eye. See the number 1 as tall, clear, and bright.

You are in a garden or a meadow. Look up at the sun. Stretch your hand up toward the sun and catch a ray of light.

Breathe out. Use the ray of light to sew up the wound. If it is deep, start deep in the wound and sew each layer until you reach the surface of the skin, where you sew the two sides of the incision together.

Breathe out. Ask all the cells around the wound to use the mesh of light to realign perfectly.

Breathe out. See the wound closed. See all signs of the wound dissolving, until the skin is once again smooth and unblemished.

Breathe out. Open your eyes, seeing this with open eyes.

To Stop Premature Contractions and Repair Placenta Previa

IF YOU EXPERIENCE premature contractions (before 37 weeks gestation), do these two exercises immediately.

CALMING THE WAVES
exercise 159

Close your eyes. Breathe out slowly three times, counting from
3 to 1, seeing the numbers in your mind's eye. See the number
1 as tall, clear, and bright.

See yourself lying on the sand on a beautiful beach,
surrounded by palm trees.

Hear the wind rustling the palm leaves . . .

Hear the waves breaking on the beach with power
and strength . . .

See the white foam.

Breathe out. Now see the waves getting smaller . . .
and smaller . . . and smaller . . . and turning into ripples.
Hear them becoming softer and softer . . .

At the same time, the wind is quieting . . .

Now hear that the waves have stopped . . .

See that the sea is as calm as a mirror.

The wind has also stopped and everything is quiet . . .

See yourself lying on the sand of the quiet, calm seashore.

Breathe out. Open your eyes.

TYING THE POUCH
exercise 160

Close your eyes. Breathe out slowly three times, counting from
3 to 1, seeing the numbers in your mind's eye. See the number
1 as tall, clear, and bright.

Imagine your uterus as an upside-down pouch with strings.

Breathe out. Pull the strings tight to close the pouch securely,
and tie a knot.

Breathe out. Tie the strings securely to a vertebra in your midback.

Breathe out. Then imagine that all the muscles of the lower
basin are like a great, golden spider web. Pull and gather each

strand of the web up high to tie them all securely to a vertebra in your midback. Tie them up to the mid-thoracic back.

Breathe out. Open your eyes, seeing this with open eyes.

Very important:

Do these two exercises every fifteen minutes until you feel the contractions have stopped.

Then continue *Tying the pouch* every hour on the hour for the next three days. Reduce to five times a day for three days, then three times a day for three days, then twice a day for three days. Then do the exercise once a day to check that your body has indeed gotten the message.

This exercise has been successful for every woman I've given it to for the last thirty-five years.

Also very important: At 37 weeks of pregnancy when the baby is viable, *untie the knot.*

To repair a condition called placenta previa do the following exercise.

TO LIFT THE PLACENTA
exercise 161

Close your eyes. Breathe out slowly three times, counting from 3 to 1, seeing the numbers in your mind's eye. See the number 1 as tall, clear, and bright.

Sense, see, and feel your mouth. Sense the inside of your lips and the inside of your mouth. Feel your gums, your teeth, your tongue.

Breathe out. Feel your tongue relaxing and dropping to the floor of your mouth.

Breathe out. See yourself becoming very small and entering into your mouth as into a domed structure. See your palate as the dome of an edifice rising higher and higher as you look.

Breathe out. Sense your uterus. See it also rising, like the dome of your mouth.

Breathe out. See the placenta as a balloon filling the domed space, allowing for lots of room for the baby to grow, expand, and move.

Breathe out. Come back to your usual size and sense, see, and feel those two similar spaces in your body.

Breathe out and open your eyes.

APPENDIX 3

List of Exercises

CHAPTER 1   PRE-CONCEPTION: CLEARING THE WAY

1. Remembering your night dream
2. Asking a question of your night dreams
3. Making your soup
4. What is my question?
5. Emptying your handbag
6. Clearing your womb
7. Cleaning your bedroom
8. Cleaning out an abortion
9. To get rid of fear
10. Manna from heaven
11. Identifying repetitive behaviors or thoughts
12. Clearing ancestral beliefs about conception
13. A tapestry of your family history

CHAPTER 2   CONCEPTION: CALLING FORTH THE SOUL

14. Take three steps back
15. Return to a place of love
16. Natural breathing
17. Repotting the plant
18. Harmonizing breath

19. Gratitude (1)
20. To call forth a soul
21. Finding the most propitious dates for conceiving
22. Shining your ovaries and uterus
23. The conception exercise
24. Meadow colors
25. Two mirrors

CHAPTER 3   FIRST TRIMESTER: EXCITING NEWS

26. Facing the needs of your dream
27. The garden of paradox
28. Going into the womb to visit your child
29. Breathing with the tree
30. Indigo column
31. Clearing color
32. The cocoon of light
33. Sweep the porch
34. Washing away fears
35. White screen
36. The chalice

CHAPTER 4   SECOND TRIMESTER: BASKING IN THE GLOW

37. Body cycles
38. Clearing catastrophic voices
39. Sweeping away bad habits
40. The dark cloud
41. To prepare for procedures
42. Color for cramping
43. Ladies' happiness
44. White petals
45. Secret garden
46. Weaving your child's life tapestry and name
47. Blue vase
48. White staircase
49. The river runs through

50. Micromovements
51. Alice in Wonderland
52. Number 1
53. Ocean of light (1)
54. Reversing
55. Ancestry support
56. Tree of life

CHAPTER 5   PREGNANCY: THE RUSH TO PREPARE

57. Freeing the inner child
58. Reversing the past
59. Taking your mother out of your body
60. The cylindrical mirror
61. TLC for yourself
62. Rehearsing the birth—the flower
63. Beuu breathing
64. Drop of oil
65. Decision making
66. The feather of truth
67. Become the water
68. Caesarean
69. Labor intent
70. Drop of oil for releasing contractions
71. Relief for fetal distress
72. Egyptian hands
73. Turning Baby
74. In the hand of the Divine
75. Ocean of light (2)

CHAPTER 6   LABOR: THE FLOWER OPENS

76. Lightening
77. Asking if the body is ready for birth
78. Free up the lower back and pelvis
79. Demeter, doorway of the mysterious feminine
80. Duck breath

81. The peach
82. Quiet place
83. Readied home
84. Immersion
85. Riding the wave (1)
86. Drop your weapons
87. Rhythm
88. Deepening natural breathing
89. Blue pathway
90. The cocooned room
91. Return to a place of love
92. The birthing dreamfield
93. Riding the wave (2)
94. White cloud
95. Elongate with the movement of the waves
96. Loosen the cord
97. Discarding
98. Rotating Baby
99. To release the placenta
100. Wound repair (1)

CHAPTER 7   POSTPARTUM AND BONDING: FIRST SMILES

101. To ease perineum swelling
102. Angelic massage for muscle aches and bruising
103. A catheter of light
104. Adrenal handles
105. Bonding with your newborn
106. Skin to skin
107. Sky in the eyes
108. Baby's name—the sound of love
109. Hand holding
110. Putting yourself in Baby's place
111. What does Baby's skin need?
112. Hatching
113. Baby as mirror
114. Turning nipples inside out

115. Timeless bubble
116. Color of your mood
117. Sighing softly, *aaah*
118. Tick tock
119. Heart coherence
120. Gratitude (2)
121. Sleep cradle
122. Grounding
123. Comforting the child inside
124. Mirror blues
125. Mirror of intent
126. The violet squeeze
127. Kegel imaginal physical
128. Mowing the lawn
129. Eye of the needle
130. Mandala in sand
131. Three fish
132. The other half of you

CHAPTER 8   FATHERS AND PARTNERS

133. To call forth a soul—for Father
134. Wounded child
135. See yourself as opposites
136. Harmonizing breath
137. The conception exercise—for Father
138. Meadow colors—for Father
139. The dark triangle
140. Magical boots
141. Plucking prosperity
142. Seeing the date your images become manifest
143. Balance male and female
144. The bridge of light
145. Father going into the womb to visit his child
146. Reversing the past
147. Father rehearsing the birth—the flower
148. Courage

149. Blue pathway—for Father
150. Beuu breathing—for Father
151. Demeter, doorway of the mysterious feminine—
    for Father
152. Drop of oil—for Father
153. Bonding with your newborn—for Father

EPILOGUE   WHEN YOUR CHILD DREAMS YOU

154. Ocean of light (3)
155. The paradox of peace

APPENDIX 1   FOR SURGICAL PROCEDURES
AND MEDICAL TESTS

156. The garden—to prepare for procedures
157. The river runs through (repeat)
158. Wound repair (2)

APPENDIX 2   FOR PREMATURE CONTRACTIONS

159. Calming the waves
160. Tying the pouch
161. To lift the placenta

NOTES

1. Kabbalah is the Jewish mystical path. Sephardic refers to the Jews living around the Mediterranean, as opposed to the Ashkenasi Jews from Eastern Europe. Colette Aboulker-Muscat (1909–2003) lived and taught in Jerusalem from 1954 until her death.

2. Genesis 12:1. Stone Edition Tanakh (New York: ArtScroll Mesorah Publications).

3. *American Heritage Dictionary of the English Language* (Boston: Houghton Mifflin, 2000).

4. Francis Crick and Graeme Mitchison, "The function of dream sleep," *Nature* 304 (July 14, 1983): 111–14.

5. K. D. White, "Salivation: The significance of imagery in its voluntary control," *Psychophysiology* 3: 196–203, in Jeanne Achtenberg, *Imagery in Healing* (Boston: Shambhala, 2002).

6. Michael Murphy, *The Future of the Body* (New York: Tarcher, 1993).

7. C. C. Kirk and D. C. Griffey, "The effect of imagery and language cognitive strategies on dietary intake, weight loss, and perception of food," *Imagination, Cognition and Personality* 15 (1995–96): 145–57.

8. G. Newshan and R. Balamuth, "Use of imagery in a chronic pain outpatient group," *Imagination, Cognition and Personality* 10(1) (1990–91): 25–38.

9. Anees A Sheikh and Charles S. Jordan (1983) "Clinical uses of mental imagery," in A. A. Sheikh ed., *Imagery: Current Theory, Research, and Application* (New York: Wiley, 1983).

10. Henri Corbin, *Creative Imagination in the Sufism of Ibn-Arabi,* trans. Ralph Manheim (London: Routledge & Kegan Paul, 2007).

11. Anees A. Sheikh, ed., *Healing Images: The Role of Imagination in Health* (Amityville, NY: Baywood Publishing Company, 2003).

12. Matthew 25:1–13.

13. Blaise Pascal, French Christian philosopher, mathematician and inventor, in his famous *Pensées*.

14. Matthew 25:1–13.

15. Psalm 39:6. Translated by Rabbi Gershon Winkler, *Kabbalah 365: Daily Fruit from the Tree of Life* (Kansas City, MO: Andrews McMeel, 2004).

16. Bereishis Rabbah, chapter 10.

17. Genesis 30:37–39.

18. Dr. Radic, Yale Department of Neurobiology, study, *Proceedings of the National Academy of Sciences*.

19. Color adapted from Dr. Dinshah's colors in Darius Dinshah, *Let There Be Light: Practical Manual for Spectro-Chrome Therapy* (Malaga, NJ: Dinshah Health Society).

20. Genesis 3:16. Bereishis (New York: ArtScroll Mesorah Publications).

21. Michel Odent, a French obstetrician who has written extensively about birthing.

22. Michael Murphy, *In the Zone: Transcendent Experience in Sports* (New York: Penguin, 1995).

23. Exodus 20:5–6. Shemos (New York: ArtScroll Mesorah Publications).

24. Isaiah 11:6. King James Translation, 2000.

INDEX

abortions
  cleaning out an abortion, 25
  clearing and repairing, 24–26
Aboulker-Muscat, Colette, x, 4–5,
  46
abruptio placenta, 135
adrenal release, 194–195
adrenaline, breast-feeding and, 213
amniocentesis, 89
amniotic sac, 68, 203
ancestors
  connecting with, 111–113
  fathers and, 255–256
  support from, 175
ancestral belief systems, 28–31
  clearing (exercise), 28–29
anemia, 99–101
annunciation dreams, 58–60
anxiety, normal (and clearing
  of), 73–76, 85–88, 246–247,
  252–253
Apgar score, 184
Assiyah (manifestation), 15, 16
athletes, visualizations and, xxvi,
  106
Atzilut (emanation), 15, 16

baby. *See also* birth; postpartum
  and bonding
  Apgar score, 184

approaching in a quiet state, 212,
  214
awareness of, 198
baby's head, size of, 158–159
benefits of being close to parents,
  197, 201–202, 203–204
chart of fetal development (week
  by week), 253
communication with, 94,
  200–208, 251–255
cries, 214–216
cries, attending to, 215–216
first stool, 209
growth rate, increasing, 281
holding, 203–204, 217
language of images and, 65
learning in the womb, 64
learning of, 200, 208
as mirror (exercise), 208
movements of, 92–94
newborn talents and abilities,
  198–202
reactions to outside stimuli, 64
seeing baby's face the first time,
  183, 252
skin-to-skin contact, 199–200,
  209
smiles, 213–214
taking care of, 203–209
time spent sleeping, 197
visualizations for, 65, 67
baby's descent. *See* lightening

backache, 105–108

balance, xxiv, 251

Bateson, Mary Catherine, 117

belief systems, 28–31, 240–241

Beuu breathing, 126–127, 182, 262–263

birth. *See also* birth options; labor; third trimester

birth plan, 129–147
  correct breathing for, 126–127
  medical model of, xiv
  Rehearsing the birth (exercise), 124–125, 155, 159, 257–259, 277–278

birth options. *See also* labor
  Caesarean section vs. vaginal birth, 134–139
  doctor or midwife, 133–134
  doula, partner, or coach, 134
  emergency hospital backup and transport, 130, 133
  epidural or no pain medication, 139–142
  episiotomy, 144–146
  fetal monitoring, 142–144
  hospital, birthing center, home birth, 130–133
  postponing cutting the umbilical cord, 146–147
  water birth, 131–132

birth rates worldwide, 6–7

birthing center, 130–133, 171–172

Black Madonna, 82

blockages
  emotional, clearing, 26–28
  removing with dream flow, 17

blood pressure, high, 101–102

bodies
  the fifth, 16
  the four, 16–17

body changes and challenges, 99–109
  anemia, 99–101
  backache, leg cramps, numbness in fingers, tingling in extremities, and breathlessness, 105–108

edema, 103–104
  high blood pressure, 101–102
  sleep disturbances, 108–110

bonding. *See also* postpartum and bonding
  for fathers and partners, 267–269
  with your baby, 195–197

brain
  exercise for calming, 71–72
  left brain, xxv, 62, 97
  right brain, xxii–xxiii, 97

Braxton Hicks contractions, 156, 261

breast-feeding, 190, 208–213
  colostrum and, 190, 209–210, 213
  consultants for, 211–212
  engorgement, 213
  exercises for, 210–212
  milk production, 213
  oxytocin and, 209

breath/breathing
  Beuu breathing, 127, 182, 262–263
  Deepening natural breathing, 170–171
  Harmonizing breath, 43, 241–242
  for labor, 126–127
  Natural breathing, 41, 101–102, 126, 170

breathlessness, 105–108

breech presentation, 135, 147

Briah (creation), 15, 16

Buddhists, 50, 242

Caesarean section, 134–139
  emergency reasons for, 136
  exercises for, 137–138, 156, 288–289
  maternal requests for, 135
  medical reasons for, 135
  safety of, 135

care for self, 82, 83, 122–123

catastrophic voices, clearing, 85–86

cell phones, potential dangers of, 78–79

cervix, thinning of, 154
Chagall, Marc, ix
Chamberlain, David, 198
children, other, integrating with
    baby, 232–233
Clearing catastrophic voices
    (exercise), 85–86
Clearing color (exercise), 72–73
clearing fears of the future, 17–19
clearing of anxiety, 73–76,
    246–247
clearing resentments, 19–35
    abortions, clearing from, 24–26
Cleaning your bedroom (exercise),
    22–24
clearing blocked emotions, 26–28
Clearing your womb (exercise),
    21–22
    Emptying your handbag
        (exercise), 20
    Identifying repetitive behaviors
        or thoughts (exercise), 29–30
    Manna from heaven (exercise),
        28
    moving past old relationships,
        19–24
    personal and ancestral belief
        systems, 28–31
Clearing your womb (exercise),
    21–22
Colette. See Aboulker-Muscat,
    Colette
colostrum, 190, 209–210, 213
communication
    harmony with, 39–40
    with your baby, 94, 200–208
    with your partner and child,
        251–255
conception, xxvii, 1–53
    calling forth a soul, 35–53,
        238–241
    changing the past and clearing
        fears, 17–19
    clearing resentments, 19–35
    conscious conception, xxvii, 7–8,
        16, 44–49, 241–242
    decision whether to have

children, 6, 7
    dreams and, 6–15
    emotions and, 49–53, 242
    father/partner's participation in,
        237–245
    four worlds and, 15–16
    harmony during, 40, 43–44, 242
    intent during, 242–245
    modern medicine and control
        over, 6
    notebooks, 9, 12, 13
    partners, harmony with, 38–44
    pre-conception (clearing the
        way), 3–33
    preparation for, 15, 16–17,
        38–44
    purification of the four bodies,
        16–17
    seminal dream, 6–7
    terminology used, xxviii–xxix
    timing of, 46–48
    visualization/imagination and,
        5–6
    voice of the dreaming body, 8–9
    waiting for, 245
conception exercises. See also
    clearing resentments
    Beliefs/belief systems, 29–30,
        30–31
    To Call forth a soul, 45–46
    To Call forth a soul—for father,
        238–239
    Cleaning out an abortion, 25
    Clearing resentments, 20, 21–22,
        22–24
    Conception exercise, 50–51
    Conception exercise for father,
        243
    Dreams/dreaming, 9–10, 10–11,
        12, 13
    Expansion, 28
    Fear, getting rid of, 27
    Harmonizing breath, 43
    Manna from heaven, 28
    Meadow colors, 51–52, 244
    Natural breathing, 41
    Repotting the plant, 42–43
    Returning to a place of love, 40
    Shining your ovaries and uterus,
        48–49

Two mirrors, 53

connection, difficulties with, 250–251

conscious conception, xxvii, 7–8, 16, 44–49, 241–242

consciousness dreaming, xxiv-xxv

courage, 260

creation, 15–16, 91

crying of baby, 214–216

decision whether to have children, 6, 7

Delphi in Greece, xix

Demeter, doorway of the mysterious feminine (exercise), 159, 263–264

depression, postpartum, 221–225

desires, 35–37
   enhancing, 51–52, 244

dialogue, xxvi-xxvii

disease states and pregnancy. *See* body changes and challenges

doctor (for delivery), 133–134

doorways, 159

Doppler (for fetal monitoring), 142–143

doulas, 134, 307–309

dream exercises
   Asking a question of your night dream, 10–11, 13
   Facing the needs of your dream, 61
   Making your soup, 12–13
   Remembering your night dream, 9–10

DreamBirth®, xii

DreamBirth (notebook), 12, 13

"DreamBirth Stories" (Rosenhouse-Raiken), 277–283

dreamfields, xxi, 197

dreaming
   as a verb, xxii-xxiii
   becoming one with your dreaming baby, 95
   consciousness of, xxiv-xxv
   in harmony with/communicating

with partners, 39–40
   history of, xix
   as interactive, xxii
   night dreams, xxii-xiii
   power of, xvii-xxix
   right brain and, xxii-xiii
   trust in, 33
   when your child dreams you, 271–275

dreams
   annunciation dreams, 58–60
   Dream Book (notebook), 9, 60
   DreamBirth (notebook), 12, 13
   as messengers from the subconscious, 59–60
   questions for, 10–15
   remembering, 9–10
   responding to the needs of, 60–62
   seminal dream, 6–7
   voice of the dreaming body, 8–9

edema, 103–104

elongation, 108

embryo. *See also* first trimester
   amniotic sac for, 68
   early development of, 58
   implantation into uterine lining, 58, 68
   placenta for, 58

emergency transport, 130, 133

emotions
   blocked, clearing, 26–28
   Garden of paradox (exercise), 63
   information from, 41–42
   paradoxical, in first trimester, 62–64
   Stepping back from (exercise), 39
   swings of, during pregnancy, 245

endorphins, 209

epidural anesthesia, xiv

epidural pain medication, 139–142

episiotomy, 144–146, 186

estrogen levels postpartum, 221

exam of conscience backward, 110

exercise, physical, importance of, 105

exercises, xxvii. *See also exercises listed after major topics*
about: summary listing by areas, 295–300
Adrenal handles, 194–195
Alice in Wonderland, 106–107
Ancestry support, 112
Angelic massage for muscle aches and bruising, 192–193
Asking a question of your night dream, 10–11, 13
Asking if the body is ready for birth, 157
Baby as a mirror, 208
Baby's name—the sound of love, 202
Balance male and female, 251
Become the water, 128, 132–133, 156, 162
Beuu breathing, 127, 182, 262–263
Birthing dreamfield, the, 174–175
Blue pathway, 171–172, 261–262
Blue vase, 100–101, 175, 197, 219
Body cycles, 83–84, 225
Bonding with your newborn, 196
Bonding with your newborn—for father, 268–269
Breathing with the tree, 69–70
Bridge of light, 252–253
Caesarean, 137–138, 156
To Call forth a soul, 45–46
To Call forth a soul— for father, 238–239
Calming the waves, 291–292
Catheter of light, 193–194
Chalice, the, 79–80
Cleaning out an abortion, 25
Cleaning your bedroom, 22–24
Clearing catastrophic voices, 85–86
Clearing color, 72–73
Cocoon of light, the, 74, 212
Cocooned room, 172
Color for cramping, 91
Color of your mood, 214
Comforting the child inside, 223–224
Conception exercise, 50–51
Conception exercise for father, 243
Courage, 260
Cylindrical mirror, the, 121–122
Dark cloud, the, 87–88
Dark triangle, the, 246
Decision making, 130
Deepening natural breathingm, 170–171
Demeter, doorway of the mysterious feminine, 159
Demeter, doorway of the mysterious feminine—for father, 263–264
Discarding, 181
Drop of oil, 127–128, 146, 181, 259
Drop of oil—for father, 264–265
Drop of oil for releasing contractions, 141–142, 156, 282
Drop your weapons, 136, 167–169
Duck breath, 160
Ease perineum swelling, 191–192
Elongate with the movement of the waves, 128, 178
Emptying your handbag, 20
Eye of the needle, 230
Facing the needs of your dream, 61
Family history, tapestry of, 31–32
Fear, getting rid of, 27
Feather of truth, the, 131
Free up the lower back and pelvis, 158
Freeing the inner child, 117–118
Garden—to prepare for an operations/procedures, 277, 282, 285–287
Garden of paradox, the, 63
Going into the womb to visit your child, 66–67, 88, 143, 253–255, 282
Going into the womb to visit your child (father), 253–255
Gratitude, 44–45, 218

Grounding, 222–223
Hand holding, 203–204
In the Hand of the divine, 149,
    167, 180, 267
Harmonizing breath, 43,
    241–242
Hatching, 207–208
Heart coherence, 217
Identifying repetitive behaviors
    or thoughts, 29–30
Immersion, 165–166
Indigo column, 71–72
Kegel imaginal physical
    (postpartum), 228
Labor intent, 140–141
Ladies' happiness, 92
To Lift the placenta, 293–294
Lightening, 155
Magical boots, 247
Making your soup, 12–13
Mandala in sand, 231
Manna from heaven, 28
Meadow colors, 51–52, 233
Meadow colors—for father, 244
Micromovements, 105–106
Mirror blues, 224–225
Mirror of intent, 226–227
Mowing the lawn, 229–230
Natural breathing, 41, 101–102,
    126, 170
Number 1, 108
Ocean of light, 109, 149, 167,
    180, 267, 273
Other half of you, 233–234
Paradox of peace, 274–275
Peach, the, 160–161
Plucking prosperity, 248–249
Preparing for procedures, 90,
    285–289
Putting yourself in baby's place,
    205
Quiet place, 163
Readied home, 164
Rehearsing the birth—the flower,
    124–125, 156, 159, 257–259,
    277–278
Release the placenta, 184–185
Remembering your night dream,
    9–10
Repotting the plant, 42–43

Return to a place of love, 40,
    173–174
Reversing, 110
Reversing the past, 118–119,
    256
Rhythm, 169
Riding the wave, 166
Riding the wave (2), 176,
    265–266
The River runs through it,
    103–104, 139, 287–288
Rotating the baby, 182–183
Secret garden, 95–96, 136
See yourself as opposites,
    240–241
Seeing the date your images
    become manifest, 249–250
Shining your ovaries and uterus,
    48–49
Sighing softly, *ahhh*, 215
Skin to skin, 200
Sky in the eyes, 201
Sleep cradle, 220–221
Sweep the porch, 75, 88, 210,
    226
Sweeping away bad habits, 87
Take three steps back, 39
Taking your mother out of your
    body, 120–121
Three fish, 232–233
Tick tock, 216
Timeless bubble, 212
TLC for yourself, 122–123
Tree of life, 113
Turning baby, 147–148, 259
Turning nipples inside out,
    210–211
Two mirrors, 53
Tying the pouch, 280, 281,
    292–293
The Violet squeeze, 227–228
Washing away fears, 76
Weaving your child's life tapestry
    and name, 98–99
What does baby's skin need?,
    206
White cloud, 177, 180, 267
White petals, 93–94
White screen, 78
White staircase, 102, 104

Wound repair, 186, 288–289
Wound repair 2, 139
Wounded child, 239–240
expansion, 27–28

false labor, 156–157, 261
family. *See also* partners
  birth and conception patterns,
    46–48
  changing your family history,
    31–32
  embracing, xxviii
  integration (postpartum),
    231–234
  the larger family, 237–269
  partners (terminology),
    xxviii-xxix
family patterns, 30
  other children and your baby,
    integrating, 232–233
  support, 111
fathers and partners, 8, 237–269.
  See also partners
  ancestors and, 255–256
  birth options checklist, going
    over with partner, 259–260
  bonding, 267–269
  as coach for birth process, 134,
    262–267
  communicating with your
    partner and child, 251–255
  conceiving consciously, 241–242
  conception, 237–245
  dreaming in harmony with,
    39–40
  during labor, 261–266
  facing the unknowns of labor,
    259–267
  fears of, 239
  harmony with, 38–44, 51–52
  inability to connect, 250–251
  inclusion in processes, 191
  participation of, 237
  partners (terminology),
    xxviii-xxix
  praise for (postpartum), 191
  pregnancy, 245–247
  pregnancy, dealing with partner's
    emotions and your own fears,
    245–247
  preparing for labor, 257–259
  prosperity, creating, 247–250
  rehearsing the birth with Baby,
    257–259
  remembering your partner's
    needs come first, 262
  role/exercises in pregnancy, 67
  supporting your partner's back,
    266, 267
fathers and partners: exercises for
  Balance male and female, 251
  Beuu breathing—for father, 263
  Blue pathway—for father,
    261–262
  Bonding with your newborn—
    for father, 268–269
  Bridge of light, 252–253
  To Call forth a soul—for father,
    238–239
  Courage, 260
  Dark triangle (clearing your
    mind), 246
  Drop of oil—for father, 264–265
  Father going into the womb to
    visit his child, 253–255
  Father rehearsing the birth—the
    flower, 257–259
  Harmonizing breath, 241–242
  Magical boots, 247
  Other half of you, 233–234
  Plucking prosperity, 248–249
  Riding the wave (2), 265–266
  See yourself as opposites,
    240–241
  Seeing the date your images
    become manifest, 249–250
  Wounded child, 239–240
fear
  during third trimester, 116–123
  of fathers and partners, 255,
    259–260
  fear of being like Father, 255
  fear of being like Mom, 118–121
  fear of not being a good mom,
    117–118
  fears of commitment, 116–117
  fears of future, clearing, 17–19,
    26

fears of losing independence, 245–246
of motherhood, 223–225
of physical closeness, 121–122
fear-related exercises
Comforting the child inside, 223–224
The Dark triangle, 246
Getting rid of fear, 27, 252–253
Washing away fear, 76
fetal distress, 143–144, 179–180
fetal monitoring (during labor), 142–144
first trimester, 57–80. *See also* pregnancy; pregnancy, exercises for
adjustment during, 70–73
annunciation dreams, 58–60
anxiety, normal (and clearing of), 73–76
defined in weeks, 58
development of embryo in, 58
ending of, 79–80
greeting your child, 63–67
morning sickness, 70–73
paradoxical feelings, 62–64
responding to the needs of your dreams, 60–62
rest, need for, 68–70
seeing your baby (sonogram), 76–79
vivid dreams during, 60
firstlings, 189–190, 201
footing, 147
four bodies, the, 16–17
fifth body (Yechidah), 16
interconnection of, 17
four worlds, the, 15–16
Assiyah (manifestation), 15, 16
Atzilut (emanation), 15, 16
Briah (creation), 15, 16
Yetzirah (formation), 15, 16
funneling, reversing, 279–280

garden
Garden of paradox, 63
Garden, the—to prepare for an

operations/procedures, 277, 282, 285–287
Gaskin, Ina May, 171, 174
gratitude (exercise on), 44–45, 218

habits, 86–87
Halek, Judith Elaine, 307
Halleck, Judith, 185
harmony
bringing bodies into, 16
harmonizing breath (exercise), 43, 241–242
with partner, 38–44, 242
reestablishing (exercise), 42–43
Hatgis, Mia, 307
hCG. *See* human chorionic gonadotrophin
high blood pressure, 101–102
homeostasis, xxiii-xxiv, 41
hormones
and baby blues, 221
for breast-feeding, 209
estrogen and progesterone, 221
oxytocin, 195, 209
prolactin, 209
hospital births, 130–133, 170–171
human chorionic gonadotrophin (hCG), 58, 68, 81

images
definition of, xx
effect on body, xxvi
imagination, xx-xxiii, 5–6, 67. *See also* visualization
imaginal field, xxv
waters of creative imagination, xix-xx
implantation, 58, 68
in-vitro fertilization, 57
inner child
Freeing (exercise), 117–118
taking care of, 239–240

Jerusalem, xii-xiii, 4
Jonas method, 48

Kabbalah/Kabbalists, 4, 15, 50, 242
Kegel exercises, 228
keloids (scar tissue), 144–145

labor, 153–187. *See also* birth options; labor exercises; postpartum and bonding
active stage of, 162, 166–167
baby's heart rate in, 280–281
"can't see straight"/"psychedelic" effects, 171
contractions defining stage one labor, 162
"crowning" in, 267
cutting the umbilical cord, 146–147, 183
early phase of, 162, 163
false labor, 156–157, 261
fathers and partners, facing the unknowns of labor, 259–267
fathers and partners, partipation of, 257–267
fetal distress during, 143–144, 179–180
fetal monitoring during, 142–144
going to the hospital or birthing center, 171–172
home birth, 172
immersion in water, 164–166
induced, 155
is baby in the right position?, 147–148, 279
lightening and engagement, 154–156, 259
making sounds, 181–182
placing baby on chest for initial exam, 183
preparing for, 124–128, 257–259
rest periods during, 163, 170, 180, 265, 266
reversing funneling, stopping early labor, 279–280
stage one: labor, 162, 163–179, 261–266
stage two: pushing and delivering, 162, 180–184, 266–267
stage three: delivery of the placenta, 162, 184–186
to stop premature contractions, 291–294
subconscious help during, 162
support during, 173, 175
three stages of, 162
transitional labor, 162, 175–179, 279
true labor, 161–187
water bag, rupture of, 161–162
welcoming baby, 183–184, 186–187
will the opening be wide enough?, 158–161
labor exercises
Asking if the body is ready for birth, 157
Become the water, 132–133, 156, 162
Beuu breathing—for father, 263
Birthing dreamfield, 174–175
Blue pathway, 171–172
Blue pathway—for father, 261–262
Blue vase, 100–101, 175
Cocooned room, 172
Deepening natural breathing, 170–171
Demeter, doorway of the mysterious feminine, 159, 263–264
Discarding (stage two), 181
Drop of oil, 127–128, 181, 259, 264–265
Drop of oil for releasing contractions, 141–142, 156, 282
Drop your weapons, 167–169
Duck breath, 160
Elongate with the movement of the waves, 178–179
Free up the lower back and pelvis, 158
In the Hand of the divine, 149, 167, 180, 267
Immersion, 165–166
Lightening, 155
Loosen the cord, 179–890

Natural breathing, 41, 170
Ocean of light, 109, 167, 180, 267
The Peach, 160–161
Quiet place, 163
Readied home, 164
Rehearsing the birth—the flower, 124–125, 156, 159, 277–287
Release the placenta, 184–185
Return to a place of love, 173–174
Rhythm, 169
Riding the wave, 166–167, 176
Riding the wave (2), 176, 265–266
Rotating the baby, 182–183
Sweep the porch, 75, 171
Tying the pouch, 280, 281, 292–293
White cloud, 177, 180, 267
Wound repair, 186
Lao Tzu, 189
Lawyer, Ruth, 308
leg cramps, 105–108
let-down reflex, 209
light, 5–6
lightening, 154–156, 259, 278
linea negra, 82
longing, 85
love, unconditional, 204
"love hormone" (oxytocin), 195, 209
Lunar Fertility Cycle, 48

Manna from heaven (exercise), 28
Meadow colors (exercise), 51–52
for father, 244
meconium, 209
medical tests, exercises for, 285–289
memories, 17–19
clearing and cleaning out, 21, 22
midwife (for delivery), 133–134
midwives, xiv-xv
milestones of pregnancy, xxvii, 55–150. See also specific

trimesters
first trimester, 57–80
second trimester, 81–113
third trimester, 115–150
moon, fertility and, 48
morning sickness, 70–73
Moro reflex, 184

naming your child, 97–99
exercises on, 98–99, 202
natural birth, 129
newborns. See baby
nightmares, 89
Nin, Anaïs, 271
nipples, 210–211. See also breast-feeding
notebooks, 9, 12, 13
numbness in fingers, 105–108

Odent, Dr. Michel, 131–132, 140
old relationships, moving past, 19–24. See also clearing resentments
orphans, 203
overdue, 154–155
oxytocin, 195, 209
epidural anesthetic and, xiv

parenting, 271–275
intuition and, 197
Ocean of light (exercise), 273
Paradox of peace (exercise), 274–275
preparing for, 38
preparing for labor, 124–128
partners, 237–269. See also fathers and partners
as coach for birth process, 134, 262–263
dreaming in harmony with, 39–40
harmony with, 38–44, 51–52
inclusion in processes, 191
praise for (postpartum), 191
terminology, xxviii-xxix

past, changing the, 17–19, 256
personal belief systems, 28–31
Piaget, Jean, 198
Pitocin, 144
placenta, 58, 81
  delivery of, 184–186
  saving, 147, 185
placenta previa, 135
  repairing, 292–294
PMS (premenstrual syndrome), 224
postpartum and bonding, 189–234
  baby blues, 221–225
  baby cries, 214–216
  baby smiles, 213–214
  being close to baby, 197,
    201–202
  bloating, 227–228
  bonding with your baby, 195–
    197, 267–269
  breast-feeding, 208–213
  eating and drinking after birth,
    190–191
  fathers and partners during,
    267–269
  fear of motherhood, 223–225
  feeling yourself after birth,
    190–195
  first four hours, 198
  first moments/firstlings, 189–190,
    201
  getting help for household tasks,
    221–222
  hormones and, 195
  integration, 231–234
  Kegel exercises, 228
  menstruation after, 229
  newborn talents, 198–202
  physical exercises, 229–230
  praise for partner, 191
  preemies and neonatal room,
    197, 203
  restructuring, 225–230
  resuming lovemaking, 233–234
  skin-to-skin contact, 199–200,
    209
  sleep deprivation, 219–221
  taking care of baby, 203–209
  taking care of your needs, 195,
    219–221

postpartum and bonding exercises
  Adrenal handles, 194–195
  Angelic massage for muscle aches
    and bruising, 192–193
  Baby as a mirror, 208
  Baby's name—the sound of love,
    202
  Bonding with your newborn, 196
  Bonding with your newborn—
    for father, 268–269
  Catheter of light, 193–194
  Color of your mood, 214
  Comforting the child inside,
    223–224
  Ease perineum swelling, 191–192
  Eye of the needle, 230
  Gratitude, 218
  Grounding, 222–223
  Hand holding, 203–204
  Hatching, 207–208
  Heart coherence, 217
  Kegel imaginal physical, 228
  Mandala in sand, 231
  Meadow colors, 233
  Mirror blues, 224–225
  Mirror of intent, 226–227
  Mowing the lawn, 229–230
  Other half of you, 233–234
  Putting yourself in baby's place,
    205
  Sighing softly, ahhh, 215
  Skin to skin, 200
  Sky in the eyes, 201
  Sleep cradle, 220–221
  Three fish, 232–233
  Tick tock, 216
  Timeless bubble, 212
  Turning nipples inside out,
    210–211
  The Violet squeeze, 227–228
  What does baby's skin need?,
    206
postpartum blues (depression),
  221–225
  Mirror blues (exercise), 224–225
preeclampsia
  Caesarean birth for, 135
  swelling as sign of, 104
pregnancy. See also specific

trimesters
as big business, xiii–xiv
body challenges (diseases) in,
99–109
father's role in, 67, 245–247
fears about, 245–246
first trimester, 57–80
letting your practitioner know
your preferences, 129
milestones of, xxvii
a personal experience, ix–x
second trimester, 81–113
test sticks for, 58–59
third trimester, 115–150
your birth plan/options, 129–147
pregnancy: exercises for first
trimester
Breathing with the tree, 69–70
The Chalice, 79–80
Clearing color, 72–73
Cocoon of light, 74
Facing the needs of your dream,
61
Garden of paradox, 63
Going into the womb to visit
your child, 66–67, 253–255,
282
Indigo column, 71–72
Sweep the porch, 75
Washing away fears, 76
White screen, 78
pregnancy: exercises for second
trimester
Alice in Wonderland, 106–107
Ancestry support, 112
Blue vase, 100–101
Body cycles, 83–84
Clearing catastrophic voices,
85–86
Color for cramping, 91
Dark cloud, 87–88
Going into the womb to visit
your child, 66–67, 88, 253–
255, 282
Ladies' happiness, 92
Micromovements, 105–106
Number 1, 108
Ocean of light, 109
Preparing for procedures, 90

Reversing, 110
The River runs through it,
103–104, 139
Secret garden, 95–96
Sweep the porch, 88
Sweeping away bad habits, 87
Tree of life, 113
White petals, 93–94
White screen (for amniocentesis),
78
White staircase, 102, 104
Your child's life tapestry and
name, 98–99
pregnancy: exercises for third
trimester
Become the water, 128, 132–133
Beuu breathing, 127, 263
Caesarean, 137–138
Cylindrical mirror, 121–122
Decision making, 130, 133
Drop of oil, 127–128, 141–142,
146, 259, 264–265
Egyptian hands, 145–146
Elongate with the movement of
the waves, 128, 178–179
Feather of truth, 131, 133
Freeing the inner child, 117–118
In the Hand of the divine, 149,
167
Labor intent, 140–141
Ocean of light, 149
Rehearsing the birth—the flower,
124–125, 155, 257–259,
277–278
Relief for fetal distress, 143–144
Reversing the past, 118–119,
256
The River runs through it,
103–104, 139
Taking your mother out of your
body, 120–121
TLC for yourself, 122–123
Turning baby, 147–148, 259
Wound repair 2, 139
premenstrual syndrome (PMS), 224
progesterone levels postpartum,
221
prolactin, 209
prosperity, creating, 247–250

Plucking prosperity (exercise), 248–249

Seeing the date your images become manifest (exercise), 249–250

questions for your night dreams, 10–15

quickening, 92–94

Raiken, Claudia. *See* Rosenhouse-Raiken, Claudia

rape, 136

religions, xviii

repetitive behaviors or thoughts (exercise), 29–30

resentments. *See* clearing resentments

rest
  necessity of, 68–70, 96
  need for in first trimester, 68–70

resting with attentiveness, 94–96

restructuring after birth, 225–230

right brain, xxii-xiii, 97

Rosenhouse-Raiken, Claudia, x, xi-xii, 308
  excerpts of dreambirth stories by, 277–283

Salk, Lee, 217

Sandburg, Carl, 3

Sarah and Abraham (Biblical story), xviii

Schiff, Jackie, 308

second trimester, 81–113. *See also* pregnancy; pregnancy, exercises for
  body challenges in, 99–109
  body changes in, 82–84, 99–109
  defined in weeks, 58
  let yourself be cared for, 82, 83
  naming your child, 97–99
  questions about your child, 97–99
  quickening, 92–94
  reality and worries, 84–88

resting and immersion, 94–96
  support, 111–113
  testing, coping with, 88–92

Secret, The, 36

segregation, racial, 28

self-care, 195, 219–221

seminal dream, 6–7

Shainberg, Catherine, 305

shoulder presentation, 147

sleep
  after the birth, 194
  deprivation after the birth, 219
  disturbances during pregnancy, 108–110
  having baby sleep with your, 219
  postpartum sleep deprivation, 219–221

Sleep cradle (exercise), 220–221

smiles, 189–234
  baby smiles, 213–214

sonograms, 76–79
  protection exercise for, 77–78
  recommendations for, 77
  safety questions, 77

soul
  calling forth a soul, 35–53, 238–241, 245

spirit image, 242

spinal issues and health, 105–108

spirit body, 50, 242

spirit doll, xi

spirit womb, 57

spiritual traditions, xviii

sports therapy, visualizations and, xxvi

Stern, Izetta, 309

still small voice, 8–9

stress, 73–76

subconscious, xviii, 84, 120, 156
  belief systems and, 30
  dreams as messengers from, 59–60
  as non-linear, xxviii

support, 111–113
  during labor, 173

surgical procedures and medical
tests, 285–289
    The Garden—to prepare for
        procedures, 285–287
    The River runs through,
        287–288
    Wound repair 2, 288–289
surrogate mothers, 57
swelling (edema), 103–104

Tao Tse Ching, 153
Tarot cards
    The Devil, 37–38
    The Lovers, 36, 37
testing, coping with, 88–92,
    285–289
    Color for cramping (exercise), 91
    Prepare for procedures (exercise),
        90, 282
    waiting for results, 91
third trimester, 115–150. See
    also birth options; pregnancy;
    pregnancy, exercises for
    becoming a mom, 116–123
    birth plan/options, 129–147
    defined in weeks, 58
    fears during, 116–123
    is baby in the right position?,
        147–148, 279
    letting your practitioner know
        your preferences, 129
    perineal massage, 145–146
    preparing for labor, 124–128
    trusting the process, 148–150
tingling in extremities, 105–108
Tomatis, Alfred, 199
training group for birth
    professionals, x-xii
transverse presentation, 135, 147
trust yourself, 12, 33, 88
trusting the process, 148–150

ultrasound imaging. See sonograms
umbilical cord
    cutting of, 183
    postponing cutting of, 146–147
    Rehearsing the birth—the flower

(exercise), 124–125, 277–278
    saving, 147
untangling, 277–278, 278

vaginal birth
    exercises after, 191–195
    icing after, 192, 193
    vs. Caesarean section, 134–139
vernix, 267
visual effects, 171
visualization
    about your body, 84
    athletes and, xxvi, 106
    for the growing baby, 65, 67, 91,
        255
voice
    baby's recognition of, 199
    of the dreaming body, 8–9
    inner voice, 15

water, immersion in, 164–166
water bag (amniotic sac), rupture
    of, 161–162
water births, 131–132
waters of creative imagination,
    xix-xx
Watson, Nancy, 111
Welcoming Your Baby, xxviii, 151–
    234. See also labor; postpartum
    and bonding
    embracing the larger family,
        235–269
    first smiles, 189–234
    labor—the flower opens,
        153–187
    postpartum and bonding,
        189–234
    special message of, 183–184
White, E. B., 81
    "the woman who makes babies,"
        4–5
womb
    Clearing (exercise), 21–22
    Father going into the womb
        to visit his child (exercise),
        253–255

Going into the womb to visit
   your child (exercise), 66–67,
   88, 143, 282
spirit womb, 57
worlds. *See* four worlds
worries (and clearing of), 85–88

Yetzirah (formation), 15, 16

Zinser, Cynthia, 309
zone, being in the, xxv, 167

ABOUT THE AUTHOR

CATHERINE SHAINBERG, PHD, is an international expert in the use of imagery for healing physical, emotional, and mental wounds. She teaches the Kabbalah of Light, the ancient Sephardic way of inner transformation and spiritual growth, through the use of dreams, waking dreams, short guided exercises, and other techniques transmitted to her from her lineage. She founded The School of Images (SOI, a nonprofit organization dedicated to disseminating the language of imagery throughout the world) in 1982 in New York City, where she lives when she is not traveling to give workshops. She teaches internationally: privately, in groups, through webinars, and in her workshops. Her first book, *Kabbalah and the Power of Dreaming*, was published by Inner Traditions in 2005. For more information about her work please visit her website, schoolofimages.com.

DOULAS

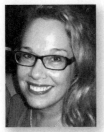

JUDITH ELAINE HALEK, CCE, CD, CHT

Director of Birth Balance since 1987, certified hypnotherapist, childbirth educator, labor doula and pre/post-natal fitness coach, Judith is a member of Catherine Shainberg's original DreamBirth® Imagery development group. She integrates DreamBirth® in all aspects of her work focused on alternative approaches in childbirth. Judith is an international writer, speaker, and filmmaker: birthbalance.com.

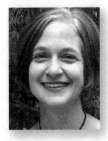

MIA HATGIS, LAC

Mia Hatgis is a New York State licensed acupuncturist and Chinese herbalist, who specializes in women's health, with a particular interest in fertility, pregnancy, postpartum, and pediatric issues. She has studied with Dr. Shainberg for over a decade, and uses DreamBirth® Imagery as an integral part of the work she does.

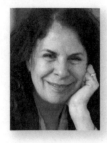

RUTH LAWYER

Ruth, originally from Colorado, now makes her home in Harlem, New York. Her work as a labor support doula springs from a longtime, sustaining love for babies and their families. The practice of DreamBirth® has had a profound effect on her life and work.

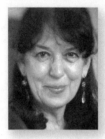

CLAUDIA ROSENHOUSE RAIKEN

Co-founder of The Birth Studio, the first center that offers childbirth education classes centered around DreamBirth®, Claudia is a childbirth educator (ICEA), a doula (ALACE), an Alexander Technique teacher and a Biodynamic CranioSacral practitioner, as well as a certified practitioner of DreamBirth®. She holds a masters from New York University in Kinesiology and Dance, and has assisted in over 250 births (as of 2012). She has seen a great increase in positive outcomes since incorporating DreamBirth® both in her work as a doula and as an educator; her respect and awe for the power of DreamBirth® is infinite.

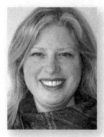

JACKIE SCHIFF, PHD, PSYD

Dr. Jackie Schiff, originally trained in New York, is now practicing in London, UK. She integrates the timeless wisdom of Torah with the practice of psychology. In Jackie's international imagery work-shops, people tap into their inner knowledge and open doors to creativity, confidence, and healing. DreamBirth® Imagery is a foundational tool of her practice, optimiz-ing birth experiences for her clients.

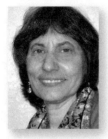

IZETTA STERN, LCSW

Izetta Siegal Stern is a psychotherapist who has worked with a full range of psychological issues and life circumstances in over 40 years of practice. She assists those facing challenges, such as infertility, loss, and pregnancy, postpartum and relationship difficulties. She enthusiastically incorporates DreamBirth® Imagery to help her clients become empowered and resilient. Izetta sees individuals and couples and is a support group facilitator for the American Fertility Association.

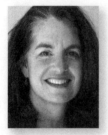

CYNTHIA ZINSER, BSN

Cynthia has been helping families through childbirth since 1986 as a registered nurse, childbirth educator, and doula. The seven years spent learning, practicing, and developing DreamBirth® Imagery enriched her life and her birthing practices, and led her to pursue a classical painting degree. In life, imagery, and art Cynthia is striving to capture and render light. She lives in New York City with her family.

ABOUT SOUNDS TRUE

SOUNDS TRUE is a multimedia publisher whose mission is to inspire and support personal transformation and spiritual awakening. Founded in 1985 and located in Boulder, Colorado, we work with many of the leading spiritual teachers, thinkers, healers, and visionary artists of our time. We strive with every title to preserve the essential "living wisdom" of the author or artist. It is our goal to create products that not only provide information to a reader or listener, but that also embody the quality of a wisdom transmission.

For those seeking genuine transformation, Sounds True is your trusted partner. At SoundsTrue.com you will find a wealth of free resources to support your journey, including exclusive weekly audio interviews, free downloads, interactive learning tools, and other special savings on all our titles.

To learn more, please visit SoundsTrue.com/bonus/free_gifts or call us toll free at 800-333-9185.

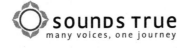